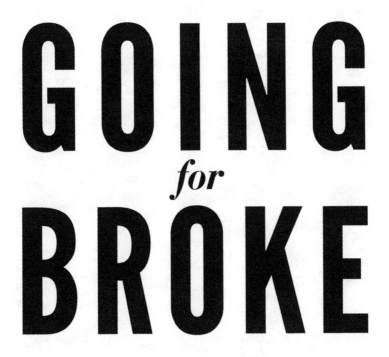

GOING
for
BROKE

DEFICITS,
DEBT, AND
THE
ENTITLEMENT
CRISIS

GOING
for
BROKE

MICHAEL D. TANNER

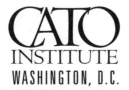

CATO
INSTITUTE
WASHINGTON, D.C.

Library of Congress Cataloging-in-Publication Data

Tanner, Michael, 1956-
  Going for broke : deficits, debt, and the entitlement crisis / by Michael
Tanner, Cato Institute.
    pages cm
  Includes bibliographical references and index.
  ISBN 978-1-939709-74-5 (hardback : alk. paper)
    1. Debts, Public—United States. 2. United States—Social policy.
  3. Medical care—United States. 4. Public welfare—United States.
  5. Welfare recipients—Employment—United States. I. Title.

HJ8119.T36 2015
336.73—dc23

2015014235

Cover design by Jon Meyers.
Printed in the United States of America.

CATO INSTITUTE
1000 Massachusetts Ave., N.W.
Washington, D.C. 20001
www.cato.org

Contents

Preface

Our growing national debt has dropped out of the headlines recently—but that doesn't mean that the problem has gone away. The "official" national debt recently topped $18 trillion and is projected to reach $26.5 trillion within 10 years. Worse, if you include the unfunded liabilities of Social Security and Medicare, our real indebtedness exceeds $90.5 trillion.

Yet despite those undeniable facts and figures, politicians from both parties continue to avoid taking serious responsibility and action when it comes to the difficult decisions that must be made. Democrats tend to believe that higher taxes, especially on the rich, can solve everything. Republicans are more likely to view spending as the problem, but they rely on cuts to domestic discretionary programs that fall far short of what is needed to really deal with the issue.

Social Security, Medicare, and Medicaid alone account for 47 percent of federal spending today, a portion that will only grow larger in the future and will increase more rapidly with the government's newest entitlement program—Obamacare. The simple truth is that there is no way to address America's debt problem without reforming entitlements.

As you read this book, I urge you to keep a couple of points in mind. First, the book focuses on our growing national debt, both explicit and implicit. It does so because debt is a particularly insidious form of taxation without representation. We reap the benefits of government spending today, while passing on the obligation to pay for those benefits to future generations that have no vote on the matter. But the reader should not lose sight of the fact that deficits and the debt are really just symptoms of a much bigger and more important problem—a government that has grown too big and spends too much.

For example, despite the focus on debt, we might actually be better off with a federal budget that spent only $1 trillion per year but ran a small deficit than we are with our current $3.5 trillion budget, even if the current level of spending was fully paid for. In theory, although probably not in practice, we could raise taxes enough to balance the budget (at least in the short run), but that is unlikely to make us better off.

Of course, if we spent less, we would likely have smaller deficits and ultimately lower debt. Indeed, my Cato colleague Dan Mitchell often points out that the only thing required to reduce the debt is for government to grow at a slower rate than does the overall economy. If government spending grows at 2 percent, while the economy grows at 3 percent, the debt would shrink as a percentage of gross domestic product.

Needless to say, government has not generally been growing slower than the economy—hence, our problem. And as spending—driven by entitlement programs—begins to rise even more rapidly in the not-so-distant future, we are only going to fall deeper in debt. Thus, debt may be thought of as the canary in the coal mine, a warning of the problems that stem from a big government growing still bigger.

Debt certainly has a cost. The Congressional Budget Office, for instance, estimates that our children will be $2,000–5,000 a year poorer because the growing debt will slow economic growth. But a government grown too large has a cost too, regardless of how it is financed.

That cost shows up first in reduced economic growth, fewer jobs, reduced take-home pay, and less overall prosperity. In an era of globalization, when Americans must compete on an international basis, taxation and regulation act as an anchor on American productivity and competitiveness. The resources that government extracts from the private sector to pay for itself are resources that are unavailable for the private sector's use in producing more goods and services. When the federal government takes money out of our pockets, we have less money to spend or save. When the federal government takes money from business, it has less money for investment, research, or workers' wages.

Second, big government undermines the "bourgeois virtues" that are necessary to a democratic and civil society. Big-government conservatives believe that government can make us virtuous. In reality, the opposite is true. When government assumes more and more responsibility for our lives, we have less and less reason to be virtuous. We are, in effect, protected from the consequences of nonvirtuous behavior. And the results are readily apparent. As government has grown, our society has become less likely to work and save, more intemperate and less concerned with the consequences of its actions, less self-reliant, and even less compassionate toward others.

And finally, and most important, big government is antithetical to freedom. Every new government program reduces our freedom just a little bit more. We are less free to manage our own lives, to decide for ourselves how to spend our money, to go into business, to plan for our retirement, to take care of our health, or to educate our children. As Ronald Reagan so correctly pointed out: "Man is not free unless government is limited. . . . As government expands, liberty contracts."

The size of the debt and its impact discussed in this book are truly frightening. But we should never forget that our true mission should always be to reduce the size, cost, and intrusiveness of government. That, ultimately, is the only way to ensure both economic growth and personal liberty.

A second point about this book is that throughout, I refer to the national debt as being roughly $18 trillion. That amount is the "official" national debt according to the Treasury Department. It is also the debt most frequently cited by the news media. As discussed within, it is derived by combining "debt held by the public" ($13 trillion) with "intragovernmental debt" ($5 trillion).

However, it should be noted that there is considerable debate among economists as to whether that is the best and most accurate debt figure to use. Many economists would prefer to use only "debt held by the public," sometimes referred to as net debt (with the $18 trillion figure referred to as gross debt). Others argue that neither figure accurately reflects the U.S. fiscal balance since neither considers the "asset" side of the ledger, such as the value of federal lands and offshore oil leases. Still others favor generally acceptable accounting principles, or some functional equivalent, under which future unfunded liabilities should be fully included.

I am satisfied with my decision to use the official debt of $18 trillion. Whatever number you choose to rely on, we can all agree that our debt is much too large.

Moreover, no one should focus too heavily on specific numbers in this book. The figures provided are the most accurate available as of January 2015, but the federal budget is a moving target. By the time you read this book, those figures will undoubtedly have changed. They won't have gotten any smaller, though.

Finally, no book like this could possibly be the work of just one person. I owe a considerable debt of gratitude to all those who helped bring it from concept to fruition. First, a great many unsung heroes contributed to the research that shows up in these pages. In particular, I would like to thank my interns Sulin Oh and Maria Iribarren, who spent countless hours at libraries, scouring the Internet, fact-checking, and meeting all sorts of my unreasonable demands.

I also want to thank John Samples, the Cato Institute's publisher, for his assistance and guidance throughout the process. Thank you, as well, to my copyeditor, Joanne Platt of Publications Professionals LLC, for turning my mangled syntax into understandable prose. In addition, I need to acknowledge Cato's crack publication team, especially David Lampo and Pat Bullock, as well as Robert Garber, our indefatigable marketing director.

Simple acknowledgment is insufficient to express my gratitude for the contribution of my research associate and collaborator Charles Hughes. Charlie's contributions are reflected on virtually every page. It is virtually impossible to overstate his importance to this project. Let me just say that without his help, this book would never have seen the light of day.

Finally, my most heartfelt thanks go to my wonderful wife, Ellen. Every step along the way, she provided encouragement, guidance, and critical review. To say that I could not have written it without her is a clear understatement. Even more important, she never stops reminding me that public policy is not about economic or philosophical abstractions but about the lives and futures of real people. That is a good lesson for us all.

1. The Coming Financial Crisis: It's Worse Than You Think

Imagine that one night you gather your family around the kitchen table to discuss your household budget. The first thing you all realize is that every week you are spending more than you and your wife are bringing in. You've simply been borrowing the rest and living off your credit cards for years. And, of course, you have nothing put away for unexpected expenses, like those remedial lessons your son will need, your daughter's orthodontics, or that leaky roof you don't know about yet.

As a result, your credit card bills now total more than your entire annual income. On top of that, you've promised to pay for your children's college education, but so far you haven't put away any money to pay for it. There's also the matter of your aging parents; caring for them will require still more time and money. Fulfilling all your future obligations will cost you thousands of dollars that you just don't have.

On the other hand, things have actually improved a bit lately. You got a small raise at work, so you are bringing home more money. And you stopped getting that morning double latte, so you've managed to slow your spending a little too. Of course, you still spend a lot more than you make, but that situation was even worse a few months ago.

So after a bit of discussion, you decide that now is the ideal time to go out and buy a new car.

If the U.S. government were a family, that's pretty much the situation it would find itself in.

Let's start with the good news. According to the Congressional Budget Office (CBO) the United States ran a budget deficit of only $483 billion in 2014. This year is projected to be even lower, just $469 billion.[1] That might not seem like such good news—we are still spending more than we take in—but it is actually a big

1

improvement. From 2009 to 2012, federal budget deficits exceeded $1 trillion per year.

Of course, we shouldn't get too excited by the improvement. Just as a family has unexpected expenditures that haven't been budgeted for, so does the federal government. Natural disasters or military actions, for example, could increase spending. So total spending in 2015 could be higher than projected.

More important, lower deficits are purely temporary. By next year, they are expected to begin growing rapidly again, particularly when vast entitlement programs like Social Security, Medicare, Medicaid, and the new health care law begin to grow more rapidly after the next decade. By 2024, deficits will again approach $1 trillion and will continue to rise in the decades that follow.

As with our hypothetical family, all that borrowing eventually adds up. For the U.S. government, ongoing budget deficits have resulted in an official national debt of more than $18 trillion as of January 2015.[2] The most recent data from 2014 showed that this debt exceeded 101 percent of gross domestic product (GDP) (the value of all goods and services produced in this country over the course of a year). For your family, that would be the equivalent of your credit card debt exceeding your annual salary.

And if you think that's bad, it only gets worse from here.

Remember that promise you made to pay for your kids' education and resettle your parents? Our government has equivalent promises. Social Security, Medicaid, and Medicare have legally promised benefits to future beneficiaries, but the government lacks the funds to make good on those promises. Trying to do so would take more money than the government has. In fact, by 2050, those three programs alone are expected to consume more than three-quarters of every dollar that the federal government raises in taxes.[3] Interest on the debt will be equal to 27 cents of every tax dollar at that point, even under an optimistic baseline scenario. As a result, nothing is left to pay for everything else that the government does, from domestic programs to national defense.

The Deficit

In 2009, our federal budget deficit hit $1.4 trillion, the largest deficit in postwar history. Since then, the budgetary situation has improved to some degree. The Troubled Asset Relief Program, which provided funding to bail out the big banks, auto manufacturers, and others, has largely been repaid. The stimulus bill passed in 2009 has mostly run its course. The sequester, imposed in 2013, has reduced the growth in expenditures and, despite being partially rolled back later that year, may continue to do so in the future. In addition, some countercyclical expenditures have declined as the recession ended and the unemployment rate declined. As a result, the budget deficit could bottom out this year at just $469 billion.

Of course, the good news is relative. Even at the deficit's low point in 2015, the federal government will still be borrowing almost 13 cents out of every dollar that it spends. Moreover, as noted above, declining deficits are just a temporary phenomenon. As Figure 1.1 shows, deficits will begin climbing again as soon as 2016. By 2024, they will approach $1 trillion and soon reach astronomical levels.

Figure 1.1
HISTORICAL AND PROJECTED BUDGET DEFICITS, 1972–2089

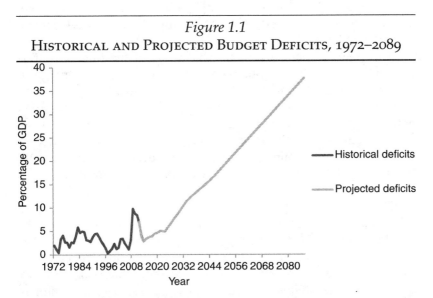

SOURCE: Congressional Budget Office, "Updated Budget Projections: 2014 to 2024," April 14, 2014; Congressional Budget Office, "The 2014 Long-Term Budget Outlook," Alternative Fiscal Scenario, July 2014.

NOTE: This uses the alternative fiscal scenario for years beyond 2024.

Looking at the deficit from another angle, federal spending has averaged 20.5 percent of GDP for the past 40 years, whereas revenues have averaged roughly 17.3 percent (see Figure 1.2).[4] Because we have been spending more than we have taken in, we have had a structural deficit equal to the difference, about 3 percent of GDP on average.

In recent years, that deficit has grown bigger. Revenues declined, reaching a low of 14.6 percent of GDP in 2010, the lowest percentage since 1950. That decline was in part due to the Bush tax cuts of 2001 and 2003 and, more significantly, to the onset of the recession in 2008. Most recently, as the economy began to recover, revenues crept upward, reaching 17.5 percent of GDP by 2014. In addition, as part of the fiscal cliff deal, the Bush tax cuts were repealed for families earning more than $400,000 per year, and a temporary two-year reduction in the Social Security payroll tax was allowed to expire. A number of additional taxes, especially those included in the Affordable Care Act, also took effect in 2013. As a result, the CBO estimates that revenues will continue to recover, eventually stabilizing at around 18.1 percent of GDP until at least 2024.

At the same time, during the final years of the Bush administration and early in the Obama administration, spending significantly outpaced revenue, leading to large annual budget deficits. However, as noted, we are currently experiencing a tiny bit of good news . . . or at least, better news. Winding down the Troubled Asset Relief Program and the stimulus spending, in combination with other efforts to restrain spending, has reduced spending in 2014 to 20.4 percent of GDP.[5] Spending is expected to grow slightly as a proportion of the economy this year, reaching 20.9 percent of GDP in 2015.

But that better news won't last. Once spending for Social Security, Medicare, Medicaid, and the Affordable Care Act really kicks in after the next decade, spending will again begin to rapidly escalate. The result will be a growing gap between revenues and expenditures, deficits the likes of which this country has never before encountered. And although no one believes that it is possible for deficits to remain on such a trajectory forever, only a fundamental change in budget policy can avert it.

4

Figure 1.2
Historic Spending vs. Revenue, Selected Years

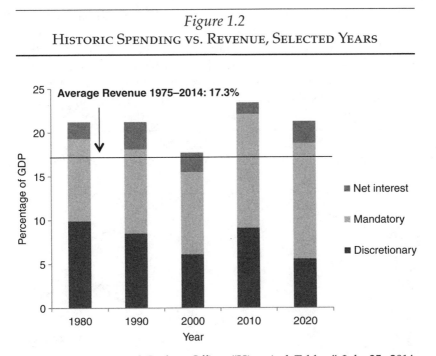

Source: Congressional Budget Office, "Historical Tables," July 25, 2014; Congressional Budget Office, "An Update to the Budget and Economic Outlook: 2014 to 2024," August 27, 2014.

The Debt

If rising annual budget deficits represent year-to-year fiscal irresponsibility, the cumulative total of that profligacy is the federal debt, which has now reached more than $18 trillion. To put that in perspective: if you earn $1 every second, it would take you a mere 573,400 years to earn enough money to pay off that debt. Or to look at it another way, that amounts to a debt of $56,496 for every man, woman, and child in America.[6] Worse, those figures capture only a portion of the actual debt we face.

The federal debt can be calculated in several ways (see Table 1.1). The U.S. government officially classifies its debt in two ways. The first is "debt held by the public," which is primarily those

U.S. government securities that are owned by individuals, corporations, state or local governments, foreign governments, and other entities outside the federal government itself. As of January 2015, debt held by the public exceeded $12.98 trillion and represented almost 73 percent of GDP, the highest percentage of the economy since shortly after the end of World War II (see Figure 1.3).[7]

Figure 1.3
DEBT HELD BY PUBLIC AND ANNUAL BUDGET DEFICITS, 1974–2014

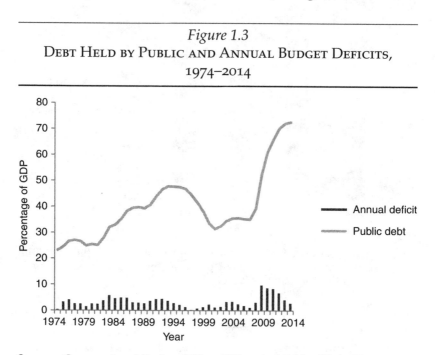

SOURCE: Congressional Budget Office, "Historical Tables," July 25, 2014.

The second classification for federal debt is "intragovernmental debt," which consists of the debts that the federal government owes to itself, such as monies it owes to the so-called Social Security Trust Fund. As of January 2015, the more than 100 government trust funds, revolving accounts, and special accounts held more than $5.10 trillion in debt.[8] The largest portion of that debt was held in the Social Security ($2.73 trillion) and Medicare ($287 billion) Trust Funds.[9] Combining the debt held by the public and intragovernmental debt produces a total federal indebtedness of more than $18 trillion.

Economists consider debt held by the public to be particularly noteworthy for several reasons. First, debt held by the public reflects government borrowing from private credit markets. The government borrowing competes with investment in the non-governmental sector, leaving less money available for private investment in such areas as factories and equipment, research and development, housing, and so on.[10] And second, interest on debt held by the public is paid in cash and creates a burden on current taxpayers.[11] In contrast, intragovernmental debt holdings typically do not require cash payments from the current budget, nor do they present a burden on the current economy.

Intragovernmental debt can also be considered somewhat "softer" than debt held by the public, since the government can control when and whether trust fund debt is repaid by, for example, altering the Social Security benefit formula. But the federal government cannot simply "write off" intragovernmental debt as inconsequential. As opponents of Social Security reform often argue, the securities held by the Social Security Trust Fund are backed "by the full faith and credit of the U.S. government." Eventually, the securities held by the various trust funds and other accounts will have to be redeemed, just as if intragovernmental debt were debt held by the public. Thus, no matter how you treat intragovernmental debt today, its repayment will ultimately have to be included in any projection of future government spending (see below).[12]

The official national debt, the combination of debt held by the public and intragovernmental debt, can be considered the equivalent of your family's credit card debt.[13] And as noted earlier, that debt now totals more than 101 percent of GDP—in other words, more than the value of our entire annual economy. For your family, it would mean credit card debt exceeding your entire annual income.

But, as bad as that situation is, it doesn't really capture the real level of debt facing this country. The reason is a third category of government indebtedness that should also be considered: "implicit debt." Like your family's unfunded promise to pay for your children's education, the government's implicit debt represents the unfunded obligations to pay promised benefits for programs such as Social Security and Medicare.

We can estimate what those obligations are, of course. We know roughly how many people will be retired each year in the future. And we know what benefits must be paid to each of those retirees under current law. We also know how much money will be available to pay those benefits, given assumptions about the number of people working, their expected wages, and the pay-roll tax rates. Unfortunately, looking at those data, we know that we will owe more in benefits than we will be bringing in in taxes. That gap is the "unfunded liability" or "implicit debt" for those programs.

Implicit debt, of course, represents the "softest" form of debt, in that there is no legal requirement to pay all the promised benefits. But "soft" does not mean debt that can be completely dismissed. Those benefit payments are called for under current law, and it would take congressional action to change them. Unless and until Congress does so, those obligations exist. That is why, for private companies, future promises to pay ben-efits are generally categorized as debt according to generally accepted accounting principles and other accounting authori-ties.[14] If the government were required to report its debt in the same way public companies do, those promises would show up as debt.

Social Security's future unfunded obligations now run to more than $24.9 trillion.[15] Medicare's unfunded liabilities are more diffi-cult to nail down, in part because of the uncertainty brought about by the new health care reform law. In 2009, Medicare's trustees estimated that the program's unfunded liabilities were $88.9 tril-lion.[16] Given the recent slowdown in the growth of health care spending though, those projections have declined dramatically to just $47.6 trillion.[17] But there is reason to be skeptical of that revised figure. The Centers for Medicare & Medicaid Services, for example, believes that the spending reductions projected under health care reform are unrealistic.[18]

Thus, the combined federal debt (debt held by public + intragov-ernmental debt + implicit debt) actually totals at least $90.5 trillion, equal to more than 500 percent of GDP (Table 1.1). If the cost-saving measures in Obamacare prove less than effective, it could be even more, perhaps as much as $130 trillion.

Table 1.1
TYPES OF U.S. GOVERNMENT DEBT

Type of Debt	Definition	Amount
Debt held by public	U.S. government securities owned by individuals, corporations, state or local governments, foreign governments and other entities outside the federal government itself	$12.98 trillion
Intragovernmental debt	Debt the government owes itself; government securities that are held by government trust funds, revolving accounts, and other special accounts	$5.10 trillion
Implicit debt	Unfunded obligations of government programs, such as Social Security and Medicare; benefits promised under current law in excess of anticipated revenue	$72.5 trillion or more

SOURCE: Department of the Treasury, "Daily Treasury Statement," Wednesday, January 8, 2015; *The 2014 Annual Report of the Board of Trustees of the Federal Old Age and Survivors Insurance and Federal Disability Insurance Trust Funds* (Washington: Government Printing Office, July 28, 2014); *The 2014 Annual Report of the Boards of Trustees of the Federal Hospital Insurance and Federal Supplementary Medical Insurance Trust Funds* (Baltimore: Centers for Medicare & Medicaid Services, July 28, 2014).

Moreover, those projections assume that interest rates on government debt remain somewhere near current levels, about 2.1 percent. The CBO points out that, even at that low rate, interest on the debt is becoming an ever-larger portion of federal spending. This year, the federal government will pay $251 billion in interest charges.[19] By 2024, those charges will rise to almost $800 billion. Not long afterward, we will be paying $1 trillion every year just for interest on the debt.[20] By 2025, in fact, interest on the debt will be tied with Medicare as the second-largest line item in the federal budget, trailing only Social Security.[21]

And that's the good news. Interest rates may not stay that low. It is estimated that every 1 percent increase in interest rates adds as much as $1 trillion in additional interest payments over the next decade. Over the past two decades, the average rate of interest on government debt has been roughly 4.4 percent.[22] Therefore, if interest rates were to return to anything close to traditional levels, trillions would be added to our future obligations.

It is also worth noting that the International Monetary Fund (IMF) warns that U.S. budget projections show a strong tendency to be too optimistic. Using its own stochastic simulation, work by researchers at the IMF suggests an 80 percent likelihood of the actual level of debt being higher than the administration's current projections.[23]

Once debt reaches the levels we are currently experiencing, it holds the potential to slow a country's economic growth. For example, the IMF looked at the relationship between federal debt levels and economic growth, concluding that from 1890 to 2000, countries with high debt levels consistently saw their economies grow at slower rates than those with low debt levels.[24]

Although it sounds ominous, debt larger than GDP is not a magic number. Still, a debt as large as we currently face potentially means fewer jobs and lower wages for American workers today. And with the debt projected to grow to astronomical levels in the future, we can expect the economy to slow further still.

That outcome should not be a surprise. In perhaps the most comprehensive study of the impact of government debt on the economy, Douglas Elmendorf, then of the Federal Reserve Board, and Harvard economist N. Gregory Mankiw listed five possible effects of increasing debt:

- An adverse effect on monetary policy, often leading to inflation and increases in nominal interest rates, with little impact on the real interest rate;
- The "deadweight loss of the taxes needed to service that debt;"
- Reduction in the discipline of the budget process;
- Increased vulnerability to a crisis of international confidence; and
- The "danger of diminished political independence or international leadership."[25]

Elmendorf and Mankiw note that not each of those effects will be experienced, nor can the magnitude of each effect be perfectly predicted, but empirical evidence has shown that some of those consequences can be quite serious and economically undesirable.

10

First, high debt levels cause inflated interest rates because potential investors demand greater returns for what they perceive as a riskier investment. As a result, central bankers may increase the money supply to counteract that effect, temporarily reducing interest rates but ultimately leading to heightened inflation (and no change to the real interest rate).[26]

Second, all money borrowed today must be repaid eventually—with interest.[27] Consequently, taxes will eventually have to be raised, and the cost to society beyond the amount of revenue raised is known as "deadweight loss." In cases of very high debt, that loss can be substantial, and policymakers would be wise to avoid fiscal policy that increases the potential for a massive burden of deadweight loss on future generations.

Third, economists, since at least the 19th century, have concluded that "government borrowing reduces the discipline of the budget process."[28] When lawmakers know that politically popular spending increases do not have to be offset by politically unpopular revenue increases, government spending tends to grow unrestrained, often for less-than-necessary purposes.

Fourth, the sheer size of the future debt could cause investors to lose confidence in the government's intention and ability to fully honor its obligations. Of course, the United States can most likely issue more debt relative to GDP than other countries because it is viewed as a "safe haven" by investors.[29] Still, the risk tolerance of investors is not unlimited.

At some point, the government would have to hike interest rates in order to continue attracting investment. The question is whether the interest rate will increase gradually over time or abruptly. In 1979, for example, with the U.S. economy weakened by stagflation, the Iranian oil embargo, and a weakening dollar, President Carter introduced a budget with deficits much deeper than predicted. International markets plunged into turmoil as the value of the dollar collapsed. Within a week, the Federal Reserve was forced to raise interest rates sharply, leading to a recession that stretched into 1982.[30]

Given the much larger debt levels we currently face, the reaction could potentially be much larger and sharper than it was in 1979.

Of course, as the CBO commented, "The exact point at which such a crisis might occur for the United States is unknown."[31] Loss of investor confidence may never happen, but it may also happen tomorrow, and there is no guarantee that the tipping point for investors is not coming soon. That is to say, although our current debt-to-GDP ratio of 101 may seem safe to investors, no one can say with absolute certainty that 105 or 110 is not the magical ratio when a sufficient number of investors bail, leaving the U.S. Treasury borrowing at much higher rates.

The danger is undeniable. As one senior Chinese banking official noted: "We should be clear in our minds that the fiscal situation in the United States is much worse than in Europe. In one or two years, when the European debt situation stabilizes, attention of financial markets will definitely shift to the United States. At that time, U.S. Treasury bonds and the dollar will experience considerable declines."[32]

Fifth, though the potential for that danger is low given the circumstances of the current U.S. economy, "the danger of diminished political independence or international leadership" resulting from a transition from a creditor nation to a debtor nation might implicate several of the aforementioned consequences, including a crisis of international confidence and loose monetary policy.[33]

In addition, the fact that roughly half of the U.S. public debt is held by foreign creditors can diminish U.S. strategic and diplomatic options. In fact, China is now the United States' largest foreign creditor, holding 10 percent of its public debt.[34] The United States has itself used such financial leverage to influence the behavior of other nations, such as in the 1956 Suez crisis.[35] It is not inconceivable that China or other countries could act in a similar way in the event of a crisis.

Finally, as mentioned earlier, government borrowing tends to crowd out private investment, because a dollar borrowed by the government is a dollar no longer available for private use. That circumstance leads to a smaller capital stock and therefore lower economic output than would otherwise be the case. If future spending were financed through debt, it would crowd out increasing amounts of private capital available for investment. As Charles Carlstrom and Jagadeesh Gokhale note: "This crowding-out effect is much larger than the effect of the balanced-budget increase in government expenditure. . . . It reflects the greater distortionary effect of the higher tax rates under deficit financing that are imposed on young and future generations to pay for the redistribution toward the initial older generations."[36]

Taking all that into account, the CBO estimates that under baseline CBO projections, real GNP per capita will be at least 2.6 percent lower by 2039 than it would be if we followed more prudent fiscal policies. Under the more realistic alternative scenario, real GNP per capita will be almost 7 percent lower (Figure 1.4).[37] That means our children will be \$2,000–5,000 poorer per capita.

Figure 1.4

DEBT DRAG ON GROSS NATIONAL PRODUCT GROWTH, 2014–2039

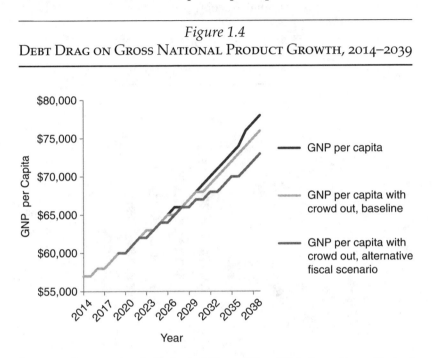

SOURCE: Congressional Budget Office, "The 2014 Long-Term Budget Outlook," August 2014, Tables 6.1 and 6.2.

Clearly, then, debt financing of future government spending would be extremely dangerous.

It's the Spending, Stupid

As frightening as those debt numbers may be, focusing on the deficit and debt is to confuse the symptom with the disease. As Milton Friedman often explained, the real issue is not how you pay for government spending—debt or taxes—but the spending itself. In other words: don't just look at the deficit, look at why we have a deficit. And the reason we have a deficit is pretty simple: government spends too much.

Some observers have claimed that recent deficits have been the result of the Bush tax cuts combined with the cost of the wars in Iraq and Afghanistan. Certainly, fighting two wars has been expensive, costing more than $1.4 trillion since 2001 by some estimates.[38] However, as Figure 1.5 shows, with the possible exception of 2007, the cost of the wars represented only a small fraction of the deficits.

Figure 1.5

DEFICITS WITH AND WITHOUT WAR FUNDING, 2003–2013

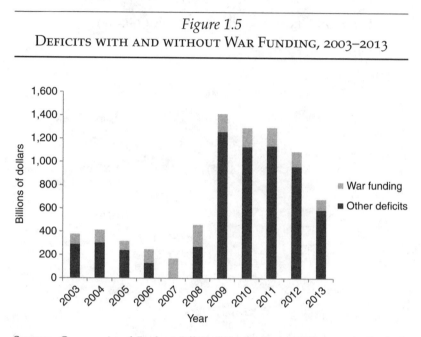

SOURCE: Congressional Budget Office, "The Budget and Economic Outlook 2014 to 2024," February 2014; Congressional Budget Office, "Historical Tables," April 15, 2014; Office of the Under Secretary of Defense (Comptroller)/Chief Financial Officer, "United States Department of Defense Fiscal Year 2015 Budget Amendment," Department of Defense, June 2014.

The impact of the Bush tax cuts is a bit more complicated, since one has to account for the dynamic impact of the tax cuts on economic growth. As the Tax Foundation points out, "no tax cut that has significant marginal rate cuts, as the Bush tax cuts did, will cost the Treasury its full 'static' score."[39]

People and businesses change their behavior when faced with lower tax rates. They invest more, work more, take more risks, and earn more money, which in turn generates additional tax revenue. That is not to say, as some conservatives wrongly claim, that tax cuts always pay for themselves. But depending on the type and structure of the cuts, tax cuts may offset part of their cost through increased growth. Gregory Mankiw and Matthew Weinzierl have estimated that the dynamic effects of tax cuts generate between 15 percent and 33 percent of lost revenue, depending on the type of tax cut.[40] A CBO report estimated that the economic effects of tax cuts would offset between 1 percent and 22 percent of the revenue loss from the tax cut over the first five years.[41]

Still, even if one accepts the most static interpretation of the tax cuts, assuming that they generated no increase in economic growth whatsoever, the tax cuts and the wars account for only a small portion of current deficits (see Figure 1.6).[42] Moreover, that estimate takes in all the Bush tax cuts, including the portion for low- and middle-income earners that was supported by the Obama administration and included in the budget deal that resolved the so-called fiscal cliff in early 2013. It also includes the cost of annual adjustments to the alternative minimum tax, which are not technically part of the "Bush tax cuts."

Figure 1.6

DEFICITS WITH WAR FUNDING AND BUSH TAX CUTS, 2003–2013

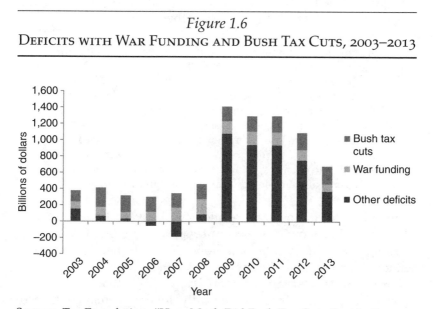

SOURCE: Tax Foundation, "How Much Did Bush Tax Cuts Cost in Forgone Revenue?" May 26, 2010; Congressional Budget Office, "The Budget and Economic Outlook 2014 to 2024," February 2014; Congressional Budget Office, "Historical Tables," April 15, 2014.

It is clear that the current budget deficit is a result of overspending, not tax cuts.[43]

Of course, some government spending is necessary. Governments must provide certain basic services, such as adjudicating disputes, maintaining police and defense functions, and, arguably, maintaining the infrastructure necessary for a functioning economy. Under a scenario with zero government spending, there would be little if any economic growth.

But beyond a certain level, nearly all economists would agree that the costs of government exceed the benefits it provides, leading to lower economic growth. For example, if government consumed 100 percent of GDP, there would be little or no economic growth. In between is a curve, with rising initial growth accompanying increased government spending, followed by declining growth once government becomes too large. Some have referred to that curve as the Rahn curve, after Richard Rahn, the former chief economist at the U.S. Chamber of Commerce (and current Cato Institute fellow), who popularized it.

As economist James Gwartney and others argue:

> As government moves beyond these core functions [of protecting people and property], they will adversely affect economic growth because of (a) the disincentive effects of higher taxes and crowding-out effect of public investment in relation to private investment, (b) diminishing returns as governments undertake activities for which they are ill-suited, and (c) an interference with the wealth creation process, because governments are not as good as markets in adjusting to changing circumstances and finding innovative new ways of increasing the value of resources.[44]

Economists debate the exact relationship between the size of government and economic growth, but few would argue that government can consume an unlimited proportion of the national economy without it having a significant impact on that economy.

For example, Harvard's Robert Barro found that "public consumption spending is systematically inversely related to economic growth," and that there is a "significantly negative relation between the growth of real GDP and the growth of the government share of GDP."[45] In other words, as government spending goes up, economic growth goes down. Similarly, Liberian economist James Guseh found that every 10 percent increase in the size of government led to a 0.74 percent decline in economic growth in democratic mixed economies, and a slightly larger 1.11 percent decline in democratic market-based economies.[46] And a study by Stefan Fölster and Magnus Henrekson of Sweden's Research Institute for Industrial Economics came to a nearly identical conclusion: a 10 percentage point increase in government expenditure was associated with a 0.7 to 0.8 percentage point reduction in the economic growth rate.[47]

A study by Prmož Pevcin of the University of Ljubljana in Slovenia found an even larger impact: a decline in economic growth of 0.15 percentage points for every 1 percentage point increase in the size of government.[48] And an older but still relevant empirical analysis of 23 member countries of the Organization for Economic Cooperation and Development by James Gwartney and his colleagues found a similar-magnitude effect: a 10 percentage point increase in government consumption as a share of GDP reduced the growth rate of real GDP by 1 percentage point.[49]

None of those studies suggests exactly where the United States would fall on the Rahn curve or how much slower our economic growth is because of the size of government. However, a U.S. government that consumes 45 percent of GDP at the federal level—and more than 60 percent overall—would clearly seem to exceed any reasonable estimate for a burden of government compatible with economic growth.

But the damage from big government should not be viewed in strictly economic terms. Much of what government does actually does more harm than good. Government social welfare programs, for instance, encourage dependency, discourage work effort, and create disincentives for family formation. Government retirement programs crowd out private savings and can leave retirees with lower levels of retirement benefits than they might have received from investing that money privately. Government health care programs can discourage innovation, decrease quality, and drive health care inflation.

As mentioned previously, the federal government currently consumes roughly 21 percent of GDP. Since state and local governments typically spend another 10–15 percent of GDP, government at all levels in the United States consumes between 31 percent and 36 percent of

GDP, far higher than what could reasonably be considered a productive level. Worse, under the more realistic alternative fiscal scenario, by 2050 federal government spending will exceed 36 percent of GDP. Adding in state and local spending, government at all levels would be consuming around 51 percent of everything produced in this country. Beyond 2050, spending continues to rise to levels that would cripple the economy (see Figure 1.7).[50]

Figure 1.7
LONG-TERM SPENDING PROJECTIONS, ALTERNATIVE FISCAL SCENARIO

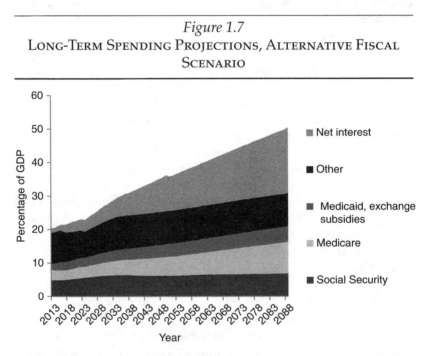

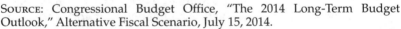

SOURCE: Congressional Budget Office, "The 2014 Long-Term Budget Outlook," Alternative Fiscal Scenario, July 15, 2014.

Regardless of the benefits, or lack thereof, from government programs, there lies the inescapable fact that unless they are cut or eliminated, all those future obligations must be financed in some way, either by a proportionate revenue increase (balanced budget) or deficit spending.[51] In other words, either government will raise sufficient revenue to cover its expenditures, or it will not.

In the end, it really is about spending.

18

Looming Tax Hikes

Financing projected levels of current and future government spending through taxes would also carry severe economic costs. Indeed, the idea of taxing our way out of debt flies in the face of fiscal reality.

Many observers suggest that we can simply tax the rich. Setting aside the simple immorality of government taking such an enormous portion of *anyone's* income, there are many reasons to be skeptical of such an approach, starting with the fact that it may not actually generate any additional revenue. It is undeniably true that in recent years some Republicans have overstated the so-called Laffer curve, suggesting that all tax cuts "pay for themselves."[52] But the basic idea behind it is simple common sense:

> Changes in tax rates have two effects on revenues: the arithmetic effect and the economic effect. The arithmetic effect is simply that if tax rates are lowered, tax revenues (per dollar of tax base) will be lowered by the amount of the decrease in the rate. The reverse is true for an increase in tax rates. The economic effect, however, recognizes the positive impact that lower tax rates have on work, output, and employment—and thereby the tax base—by providing incentives to increase these activities. Raising tax rates has the opposite economic effect by penalizing participation in the taxed activities. The arithmetic effect always works in the opposite direction from the economic effect. Therefore, when the economic and the arithmetic effects of tax-rate changes are combined, the consequences of the change in tax rates on total tax revenues are no longer quite so obvious.[53]

In other words, incentives matter. At some point, taxes become high enough to discourage economic activity and therefore produce less revenue than would be predicted under a more static analysis.

But even if one assumes that taxes can be raised without having any impact on economic growth, taxing the rich still wouldn't get us out of our budget hole—because the hole is quite simply bigger than the amount of revenue we could raise from taxing the rich, even if there were no disincentives. To put it in an admittedly oversimplified perspective: our current obligations, including both implicit and explicit debt, total almost 800 percent of GDP. The combined wealth of everyone in the United States who earns at least $1 million per year equals roughly 100 percent of GDP (see Figure 1.8).[54] Therefore, you could confiscate the entire wealth of every person earning a million dollars in the United States and still barely make a dent in the amount our country owes.

Figure 1.8
COMBINED WEALTH OF MILLION-DOLLAR EARNERS VS. U.S. DEBT

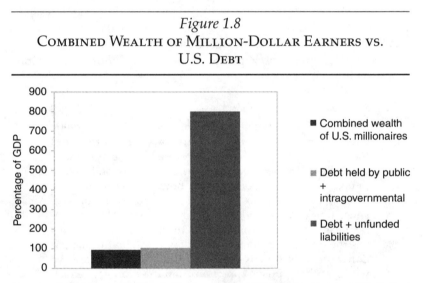

- Combined wealth of U.S. millionaires

- Debt held by public + intragovernmental

- Debt + unfunded liabilities

SOURCE: Based on author's calculations using U.S. Census Bureau, "Statistical Abstract of the United States: 2012, Income Expenditures, Poverty, and Wealth," Table 717; Internal Revenue Service, SOI Tax Stats, Individual Income Tax Returns Filed and Sources of Income, "All Returns: Selected Income and Tax Items," Tax Year 2010, Table 1.1.

Clearly, any tax increases would have to extend well beyond "the rich." In fact, the CBO said in 2008 that in order to pay for all currently scheduled federal spending, both the corporate tax rate and top income tax rate would have to be raised from 35 percent to 88 percent, the 25 percent tax rate for middle-income workers to 63 percent, and the 10 percent tax bracket for low-income workers to 25 percent.[55] It is likely that although spending as a share of GDP has declined somewhat since then, the required tax levels would be even higher today because of the accumulation of more unfunded liabilities.

Regardless of how one feels about fairness or the moral question of taxing the rich, taxes at those levels would likely slow future economic growth.

A general consensus is that some level of deadweight loss is associated with taxation, but not what the level of deadweight loss is. Estimates range from 20 percent all the way to 165 percent. The Office of Management and Budget's rule of thumb assumes that that loss is 25 percent of revenues.[56] The CBO estimates that those additional costs "range from 20 cents to 60 cents over and above the revenue raised."[57] Harvard economist Martin Feldstein points out that the actual loss from tax increases to the private sector is a combination of the confiscated revenue as well as a hidden cost of the actual increase, known as deadweight loss. That hidden cost can be very expensive. Feldstein calculates that "the total cost per incremental dollar of government spending, including the revenue and the deadweight loss, is . . . a very high $2.65. Equivalently, it implies that the marginal excess burden per dollar of revenue is $1.65."[58] That means that for every 1 percent of GDP needed to be raised in revenue, somewhere between 1.20 percent and 2.65 percent of GDP needs to be extracted from the private sector first. Most other economists use somewhat lower estimates, but, clearly, tax increases required to finance an increase in spending of more than 40 percent of GDP would place a severe burden on the private economy.

Whether we pay for future government spending through debt or taxes, we simply cannot afford the anticipated levels of government spending.

The Entitlement Tsunami

No area of government spending has been immune from overspending. Since 2000, nominal nondefense discretionary spending has increased by 80 percent, and defense spending has risen by 112—even after the sequester-imposed reductions in 2013.[59] Both defense and domestic spending will have to be reduced further if we are to begin putting our fiscal house in order.

Politicians like to pretend that you can deal with the debt crisis by eliminating "fraud, waste, and abuse" in the federal budget, and certainly there is plenty of that. But you simply cannot balance the budget by cutting the usual suspects. Foreign aid amounts to just 1 percent of federal spending. Federal subsidies to Planned Parenthood and the Corporation for Public Broadcasting amount to a combined 0.0002 percent.

In fact, all nondefense discretionary spending—everything from the Department of Education to the Federal Bureau of Investigation, from the National Aeronautics and Space Administration to the Food and Drug Administration—accounts for just 16.9 percent of all federal spending.[60] Even if every penny of such spending were eliminated, we would have still faced a budget deficit of more than $473 billion in 2012.

Defense constitutes another 16.4 percent of federal spending.[61] Clearly, cuts can—and should—be made here as well. Annual defense spending will average $552 billion over the next 10 years. By comparison, the United States spent, in 2012 dollars, an average of just $435 billion per year on defense during the Cold War (1948–1990), when we faced a much greater conventional threat. It is also important to note that that projection is only base defense spending and does not include war spending (projected to be $70 billion in 2014).[62] But no matter how deep we cut into defense and domestic discretionary spending, we will not solve our debt problems this way. That is because the true heart of rising government spending is due to entitlement programs, in particular Medicare, Medicaid, and Social Security. By 2050, those three programs alone will consume 15.5 percent of GDP.[63] If one assumes that revenues return to and stay at the 40-year average of 17.3 percent of GDP, then those three programs alone will consume almost 90 percent of federal revenues. Thus, hardly any funding would be available for any other program of government, from national defense to welfare. Adding in interest already owed would bring government spending to more than 21 percent of GDP, meaning that even a tax hike equal to nearly 4 percent of GDP would be unable to fund government beyond those three programs (see Figure 1.9).

Figure 1.9

MANDATORY SPENDING AND REQUIRED TAX INCREASE, 2050

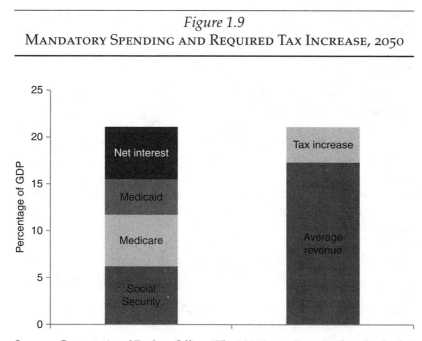

SOURCE: Congressional Budget Office, "The 2014 Long-Term Budget Outlook," July 2014.

Of course, spending is spending. Defense and discretionary spending should be cut wherever possible. But in the end, any serious plan to balance the budget long term must address entitlements.

For at least a decade, under both President Bush and President Obama, experts inside and outside government have made it clear that entitlement reform was essential to the nation's long term fiscal health. Most recently, in December 2010, the bipartisan National Commission on Fiscal Responsibility and Reform warned that we have reached a "moment of truth" for budget reform.[64]

If anything, those warnings—over many years and across political and ideological differences—have understated the threat to future generations. But so far, both political parties have sought partisan political advantage rather than dealing with the looming threat. Democrats demagogued President Bush's attempts to reform Social Security and continue to attack any Republican who raises the issue.[65] Republicans criticized Democrats for daring to make cuts, however tentative, in Medicare as part of their health care reform effort.[66] This situation must change.

Conclusion

If your family faced unpaid bills, mounting debt, and enormous unfunded future obligations but decided to keep spending money as if you had no problem, you might justifiably be called irresponsible. Yet our country's political leaders behave just as irresponsibly.

Our nation faces a massively growing debt that threatens our economic future. But as bad as that debt is, it is merely a symptom of a larger disease: a rapidly growing government that is consuming an ever-larger share of our national economy. Unless decisive action is taken, government at all levels in the United States will consume roughly 60 percent of GDP by the middle of the century and will rise to unimaginable levels thereafter. A government of that size is a threat not just to economic growth but to our liberty and our way of life.

Our looming fiscal train wreck has been amply abetted by both political parties. But unless the United States learns to live within its means, a true economic disaster beckons. That means Congress is going to have to cut spending at all levels. Both discretionary and defense spending will have to be scrutinized and pared back to affordable—not to mention constitutional—levels.

But no meaningful effort to control the size and cost of the federal government can occur without dealing with entitlement spending, in particular by restraining and reforming Medicare, Medicaid, and Social Security. Continuing to duck entitlement reform may well be "politically convenient," but doing so will condemn our children and our grandchildren to a world of mounting debt and higher taxes.

That reform must go beyond mere tinkering; it must restructure the programs in fundamental ways. The following chapters will examine those programs in more detail and suggest ways that such reforms could happen.

2. Is the United States Becoming Greece?

The United States is hardly unique in facing a mounting debt crisis. Although Europe's debt crisis has faded from the headlines as the economic recovery has taken hold, it remains clear that the modern welfare state is unsustainable, facing fiscal catastrophe, stagnating economic growth, punishing taxes, and prolonged joblessness. Although the immediate crisis (with the exception of Greece) has been postponed, European countries have nonetheless been forced, kicking and screaming, to rethink their approach to social welfare.

The Greek, Irish, and Portuguese governments alone owe some €751 billion (roughly $900 billion). Spain owes more than those three combined, €1.012 trillion, while Italy and France each owe more than €2 trillion. All told, European Union (EU) countries owe more than €11.93 trillion.[1] And that is just the debt that appears "on the books." If one includes the unfunded liabilities of their pension and health care systems, Europe is well over €100 trillion in debt.

Europe's debt problems have generated enormous economic and social instability. Indeed, the fate of the euro itself has become uncertain. The ultimate fallout is likely to be worldwide, including a continued slowing of U.S. economic growth.

Europe's ongoing debt crisis provides an extraordinary laboratory, enabling us to view the results once the modern welfare state becomes wholly unaffordable. The instability being seen in Europe today presents the likely endpoint for the United States, unless we are able to put our economic house in order. The key question is, how far has the United States traveled down the road toward a European-style debt crisis?

Europe's Debt Crisis

Both short-term budget deficits and long-term debt have reached crushing levels in nearly all EU countries. In 2013, the average EU nation ran a deficit equal to 3.2 percent of its gross domestic product (GDP), but many countries faced much bigger shortfalls.[2]

As bad as annual budget deficits are, national debts are worse, averaging 87 percent of GDP. Greece, Ireland, Italy, and Portugal have national debts in excess of 115 percent of their GDP, with Belgium (105.1 percent) and Cyprus (111.7 percent) close behind.[3] In all, 14 European countries have debt ratios higher than the 60 percent of GDP mandated by the Maastricht Treaty that created the eurozone: Austria, Belgium, France, Germany, Great Britain, Greece, Hungary, Ireland, Italy, Malta, the Netherlands, and Portugal were joined by Cyprus and Spain. Croatia, which became the 28th EU member country in July 2013, is already well above the 60 percent ratio.[4]

It could be argued, of course, that a significant portion of that debt is due to the recession, which both drove down economic growth and revenues and increased countercyclical spending. Programs such as unemployment insurance and income support measures naturally spend more during an economic slowdown. In addition, most nations undertook various Keynesian stimulus measures to spur growth, although those stimulus measures were more limited than those in the United States (see below). And several nations, notably Ireland and Spain, intervened to bail out their banking sectors. As a result, publicly held debt was 40 percent higher, on average, by 2013 than before the recession began.[5] As those programs end and economic growth resumes, debt-to-GDP ratios will likely decline in the short term. If so, countries are not as close to their debt limits as a real-time snapshot would seem to indicate.

However, it should be noted that most European countries had a substantial debt load even before the recession. Debt-to-GDP ratios in countries that now make up the EU are generally higher today than they were at the end of the Great Depression, although crisis-related factors were similar. That fact suggests that the current debt levels cannot simply be blamed on the recession; countries started the current crisis in a much weaker debt position.[6] That previous debt meant that when those countries reacted to the recession with Keynesian stimulus spending, they were adding debt upon debt. It also means that even if countries can reduce their debt to prerecession levels, they will still be in a perilous financial condition.

Moreover, most published reports on the size of Europe's debt understate the problem. That is because they consider only one type of debt, "debt held by the public," which is primarily those government securities owned by individuals, corporations, foreign governments, and other entities. However, as discussed in Chapter 1, debt held by the public captures only a small portion of a nation's real debt. A country's actual level of indebtedness, or fiscal imbalance, therefore, is better considered as the difference between the cost of continuing current government spending programs, including promised benefits under pension and health care programs, as well as existing public (and intragovernmental) debt, minus anticipated tax revenues. A country's total indebtedness or fiscal imbalance is the gap between future spending and future revenue embedded in current fiscal policies.

For instance, although Great Britain's "official" debt is roughly £1.5 trillion, an all-time high, its actual debt is as much as £5 trillion.[7] If Britain hopes to meet all its future obligations, it would need to have an additional £5 trillion on hand today that it could invest at standard interest rates.

The real indebtedness of most European countries is several times larger than the value of all goods and services produced in those countries over the course of a year (GDP). Britain owes 333 percent of its annual GDP, but that is actually better than most of its peers; France, for instance, has unfunded liabilities in excess of 549 percent of GDP; not surprisingly, Greece is in the worst trouble of any country not facing a post–Soviet era debt, with unfunded obligations in excess of 875 percent of its GDP.[8]

Even measured against total future GDP, European debt burdens are enormous, averaging almost 10 percent of all future economic output.[9] That amount would be, of course, on top of current levels of government consumption, which could reasonably be expected to continue.

But is the United States appreciably better off?

Comparison of the U.S. and European Debt Burdens

As Figure 2.1 shows, the U.S. budget deficit actually looks pretty good compared with most European countries, with a deficit lower than most of the major economies besides Germany. However, it is important to recall that as recently as 2012, we were running a deficit equal to 7 percent of our GDP, a larger deficit as a percentage of GDP than any EU country except for Greece, Ireland, and Spain. Our budget deficit has since fallen to the point it is now—which is also lower than France, Portugal, Ireland, Spain, Greece, Slovenia, and the United Kingdom—but remains above the EU average, in part because smaller countries like Estonia, Latvia, and Luxembourg lower the average budget deficit in the EU.

Figure 2.1
ANNUAL BUDGET DEFICITS OF SELECTED COUNTRIES, 2013

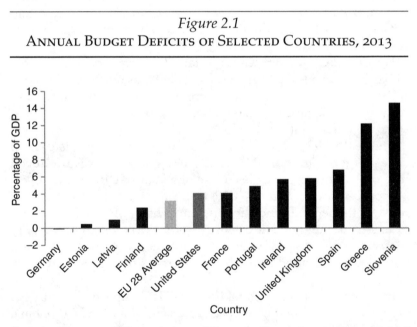

SOURCE: European Commission, "General Government Gross Debt," Eurostat Database.

Although our relatively low deficit is good news, one should remember that it is a temporary phenomenon. More important, our $18 trillion national debt doesn't look nearly as good. Compared with EU countries, the U.S. national debt is larger, as a percentage of GDP, than that of all but five EU nations: Greece and Ireland again, as well as Belgium, Italy, and Portugal (Figure 2.2).

Figure 2.2
GOVERNMENT DEBT OF SELECTED COUNTRIES, 2013

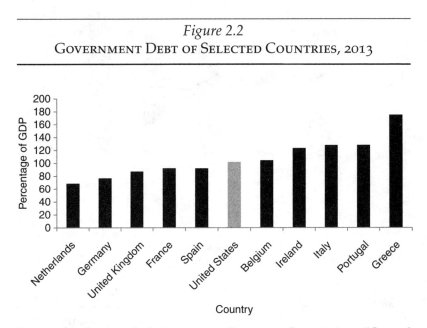

SOURCE: Author's calculations using European Commission, "General Government Gross Debt," Eurostat Database; Federal Reserve Bank of St. Louis, "Federal Debt: Public Debt as Percent of Gross Domestic Product," Federal Reserve Economic Data.

Or consider this: our national debt amounts to roughly $55,719 per person (see Figure 2.3). That means that every American man, woman, and child owes more than the citizens of any EU country.[10]

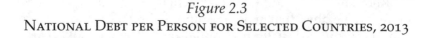

Figure 2.3

NATIONAL DEBT PER PERSON FOR SELECTED COUNTRIES, 2013

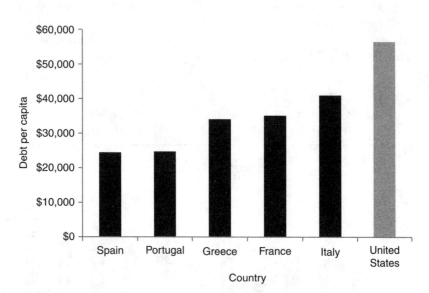

SOURCE: Author's calculations using European Commission, "General Government Gross Debt," Eurostat Database; European Commission, "Population on 1 January," Eurostat Database; Department of the Treasury, "Daily Treasury Statement: January 8, 2014."

As was discussed in Chapter 1, to truly appreciate a country's debt, we also need to consider the "implicit debt" or the unfunded obligations of pension and health care programs, that is, the benefits promised under those programs in excess of anticipated revenues. As we have seen, for the United States, as for most countries, such implicit debt dwarfs the explicit debt. The real U.S. indebtedness— taking into account both explicit and implicit debt—actually totals at least $90.5 trillion, but it could be much more if the cost constraints in Obamacare ultimately prove ineffective.

Measuring that total indebtedness against similar measures for other countries shows just how bad the U.S. situation potentially is. Even under the best-case scenario, the United States is deeper in debt than Ireland, Italy, Spain, or the United Kingdom.

Calculating the proportion of a country's future GDP stream that will be required to finance future debt does not provide any brighter a picture. As Figure 2.4 shows, the average European country will have to spend 9.9 percent of its GDP every year—forever—just to pay for its debt. That's bad, but the United States is in a position almost as dire. We face a debt equal to 9 percent of our future GDP stream. For your family, that's the equivalent of having to pay an additional 9 percent of your before-tax income for the rest of your life just to pay off your debt.

Figure 2.4
PERCENTAGE OF FUTURE GDP NEEDED TO PAY DEBT IN THE UNITED STATES (2012) AND SELECTED EUROPEAN COUNTRIES (2010)

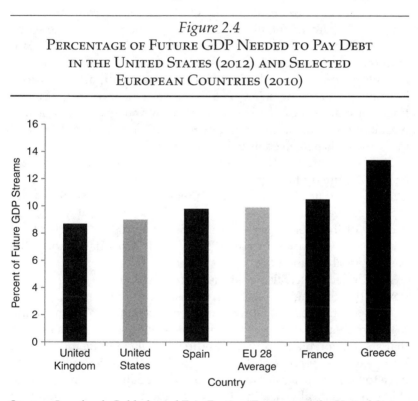

SOURCE: Jagadeesh Gokhale and Erin Partin, "Europe and the United States: On the Fiscal Brink?" *Cato Journal* 33, no. 2 (Spring–Summer 2013): 193–210.

The slow economc growth that the United States has seen coming out of the recession may be evidence that we are already seeing some consequences from our debt overhang. However, if we have not yet suffered the consequences of such debt in the same way as Europe, it is because the United States has certain economic advantages that have shielded us so far. The first of those advantages is the simple size of the U.S. economy. U.S. GDP is nearly 50 percent greater than that of China, the world's second-largest economy, and not much less than the combined GDP of all 28 EU nations. That factor allows the U.S. to absorb more debt than smaller economies.

Second, the U.S. dollar remains the world's reserve currency, representing roughly 62 percent of the world's reserves, compared with roughly 26 percent for the euro.[11] As the Congressional Research Service notes: "Investors may be willing to give up a significant amount of return if an economy offers them a particularly low-risk repository for their funds. The United States, with a long history of stable government, steady economic growth, and large, efficient financial markets, can be expected to draw foreign capital for this reason."[12] The risk of inflation, devaluation, or default on U.S. debt instruments is perceived as being relatively low.

The deterioration of Europe's fiscal situation has actually strengthened the United States' position as a "safe haven" for investment. The reason is not because of any strength or improvement to the U.S. fiscal balance, which has grown worse in recent years, but because of the even more rapid increase in European debt and the accompanying market turmoil. The United States has become the best of possible bad options.

The United States also controls its own currency, giving it more flexibility in managing short-term economic fluctuations.

As a result, investors, both at home and abroad, have been willing to lend money at extremely attractive rates. But we should not assume that such favorable borrowing conditions will continue indefinitely. If there were a loss of confidence in U.S. debt, the government would have to hike interest rates in order to continue attracting investment. Without specifically naming Greece or the EU, the Congressional Budget Office (CBO) nevertheless warns: "As other countries' experiences show, it is also possible that investors would lose confidence abruptly and interest rates on government debt would rise sharply. The exact point at which such a crisis might occur for the United

States is unknown, in part because the ratio of federal debt to GDP is climbing into unfamiliar territory."[13]

Over the past two decades, the average rate of interest on government debt has actually been 4.4 percent.[14] If interest rates were to return to anything close to traditional levels, they would add trillions to our future obligations. For example, according to the CBO, if the interest rates rose to their 1991–2000 levels, net interest payments would be higher in each year by amounts rising from $13 billion in 2014 to $274 billion in 2023. From 2014 through 2023, total interest costs would be higher by more than $1.44 trillion.[15]

Should U.S. interest rates spike, we could easily find ourselves facing a similar death spiral. However, in our case, there is no outside entity capable of intervening.

In 1979, for example, when the U.S. economy was pummeled by stagflation, the oil embargo, and a weakening dollar, President Carter introduced a budget with deficits much deeper than had been predicted. International markets plunged into turmoil as the value of the dollar collapsed. Within a week, the Federal Reserve was forced to raise interest rates sharply, leading to a recession that stretched into 1982.[16] Given the much higher debt levels we currently face, the reaction could be much larger and sharper than it was in 1979. The CBO warns that such a spike in interest rates would lead to huge losses for bondholders, possibly precipitating a major economic crisis that "could cause some financial institutions to fail."[17]

To see how close the danger is, one need only look to recent declines in the U.S. credit rating. In 2011, Standard and Poor's downgraded the United States from AAA to AA+. That downgrading now puts the U.S. creditworthiness in the same category as France, Guernsey, and the Isle of Man, and below that of such countries as Australia, Finland, and Liechtenstein.[18]

The Burden of Big Government

On average, governments (at all levels of government) in EU countries today consume almost 45 percent of their GDP. Spending by the federal government in the United States amounted to 20.8 percent of GDP in 2013, well below European averages, though well above historical U.S. averages. However, if one includes state and local spending, total government spending in the United States reaches roughly 31 percent of GDP, creeping a bit closer to European levels. Worse, under the more realistic alternative fiscal scenario, by 2050 federal government spending will exceed 36 percent of GDP. Adding in state and local spending, government at all levels would be consuming around 51 percent of GDP, roughly comparable to the burden of government that we associate with Europe (see Figure 2.5).[19]

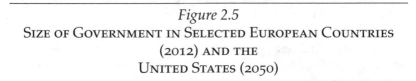

Figure 2.5
SIZE OF GOVERNMENT IN SELECTED EUROPEAN COUNTRIES
(2012) AND THE
UNITED STATES (2050)

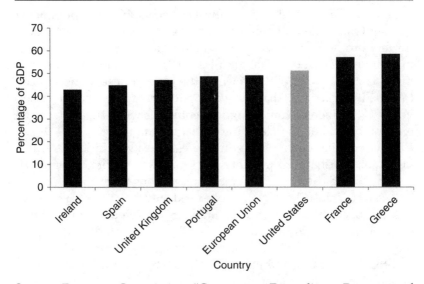

SOURCE: European Commission, "Government Expenditure, Revenue and Main Aggregates." Eurostat Database; Congressional Budget Office, "The 2014 Long-Term Budget Outlook," July 2014.

The United States has long been accustomed to an economy that grows faster than those in Europe. That is one reason why our unemployment rate has been much lower. However, if the United States ends up with a European-size government, we can expect to see slower European levels of growth, and much higher, European-level unemployment.

Conclusion

The United States faces a massively growing debt that threatens our economic future. But as bad as that debt is, it is merely a symptom of a larger disease: a rapidly growing government that is consuming an ever-larger share of our national economy. The United States is well down the road toward a debt crisis similar to Europe's. That we haven't already experienced such a crisis is the fortuitous result of the U.S. position as the world's reserve currency combined with the overall strength of our economy. But that factor will not protect us forever.

Unless the United States learns from the failure of Europe's welfare state and acts now to reduce spending, to reform entitlements, and to reduce the growing burden of government, we will eventually find ourselves in the same situation as Greece.

3. The Debt Deniers

Unsurprisingly, given the political divisions in this country, not everyone agrees with the analysis shown in the first two chapters. Think of your irrepressible—and irresponsible—Uncle Paul, who on hearing that you are worried about your family's debt, tells you to relax; tomorrow will take care of itself, things are not as bad as you think, worrying is for suckers, and so on. So too, do some regard the national debt.

Indeed, in recent years, a virtual cottage industry has developed among pundits and politicians who deny that the United States is facing a debt crisis. Paul Krugman, for example, pronounces the debt problem—or at least the deficit—"mostly solved."[1] While still at *Slate*, Matt Yglesias asked, "What sovereign debt crisis? There certainly isn't one in the United States."[2] Bruce Bartlett, every liberal economist's favorite former conservative, adds that "our long-term budget situation is not nearly as severe as even many budget experts believe."[3]

Debt deniers come from a variety of perspectives and offer a variety of critiques. Some suggest that government debt is simply not a problem. Others concede that debt can be bad but argue that it can serve a beneficial purpose during times of economic distress. Still others are opposed to too much debt in the abstract but suggest that the U.S. debt crisis is not actually as severe as has been predicted. Regardless of their approach, all oppose the sorts of actions called for in this volume, such as significant reductions in federal spending or major reform of entitlement programs.

The debt deniers have a great deal of influence in the media and on Capitol Hill. Given the already powerful institutional barriers to dealing with the debt, it is important to understand and rebut the arguments made by those who claim that we have no debt crisis.

The Debt Deniers' Rationales

Those rejecting the seriousness of our growing national debt offer several rationales for their position.

We Owe It to Ourselves

Perhaps the most fundamental question is whether the level of debt that a country owes is important in the first place. After all, John Maynard Keynes maintained that during times of recession, "the whole of the labor of the unemployed is available to increase the national wealth. It is crazy to believe that we shall ruin ourselves financially by trying to find means for using it and that safety lies in continuing to maintain idleness."[4]

That statement is a bit of an oversimplification of Keynes's position, since he actually believed that governments should run surpluses during times of economic prosperity. Although he believed that government debt could be a countercyclical force for economic growth (see next section), he wasn't really an advocate of unconstrained debt.

Still, some economists continue to make that Keynesian argument. Paul Krugman writes: "People think of debt's role in the economy as if it were the same as what debt means for an individual: there's a lot of money you have to pay to someone else. But that's all wrong; the debt we create is basically money we owe to ourselves, and the burden it imposes does not involve a real transfer of resources."[5]

As is illustrated by Krugman's statement, the core of that line of reasoning rests on three assumptions:

- It is incorrect to draw an analogy between private and public debt;
- Public debt does not involve any transfer of burden to future generations; and
- There is an important distinction between an internal and an external public debt.[6]

Essentially, advocates of the "we owe it to ourselves" school are arguing that debt merely causes a transfer of resources from taxpayers to bondholders. To the degree that those bondholders are also Americans, even if our children have to pay off our debt in the future, they will be paying it only to other members of their generation. Thus, that generation will, on net, be no poorer because of the debt created by their parents.

Think of it this way. If you lend money to your wife, your family is no poorer. The same holds true when she pays you back.[7]

Even interest payments do not represent an actual loss of wealth, according to that line of reasoning, since they remain within the broader economy.

That reasoning is not entirely incorrect. But it is a mistake to think in terms of "the economy" or "the generation," as a unified whole, rather than an aggregation of distinct individuals. As James Buchanan has pointed out, even within the boundaries of a country, the holder of government debt may not be the individual who ultimately must pay the taxes that pay the interest or principal. The payer and payee are separate entities. For example, Mr. Jones holds a government bond. But Mr. Smith pays the taxes that pay interest to Mr. Jones. They are not the same person just because both happen to be Americans.[8]

When thinking about debt, there are effectively three different players: bondholders, current taxpayers, and future taxpayers. All have different interests and expectations. The bondholder, for instance, is not concerned about the use of his funds once he has received the bond. Even if the money he has lent the government is wasted, generating little or no increase in overall wealth, he is still guaranteed income in the future, from both interest and the repayment of principal, so he is not bearing the burden of debt creation. Similarly, current taxpayers bear little burden since they are not paying directly.

The burden therefore rests on future taxpayers—our children and grandchildren. Or as Ludwig von Mises explained: "The fact is that the public debt embodies claims of people who have in the past entrusted funds to the government against all those who are daily producing new wealth. It burdens the producing strata for the benefit of another part of the people."[9]

Keynesians would respond by suggesting that we should also account for the degree to which the future taxpayer benefits from the spending funded through debt. As Buchanan explains,

"If the debt is created for productive public expenditure, the benefits to the future taxpayer must, of course, be compared with the burden so that, on balance, he may suffer a net benefit or a net burden."[10]

In other words, if the borrowed money were used, say, to build a road that increased productivity and therefore economic growth, the future taxpayer may be wealthier than he would have been in the absence of that road. A full accounting of transfers should take that into account.

However, to the extent that the borrowing funds current transfer payments or other nonproductive spending, it generates no gains for future taxpayers, leaving them to bear the full burden. As Buchanan explains: "[The future taxpayer] now must reduce his real income to transfer funds to the bondholder, and he has no productive asset in the form of a public project to offset his genuine *sacrifice*. Thus, the taxpayer in future time periods, that is, the future generation, bears the full primary real burden of the public debt."[11]

Only a tiny fraction of government spending can be considered investment of the type that generates net future gains. By some estimates, in fact, only around 15 percent of federal spending can be considered an investment, even using a broad definition of the term that includes "human investment," such as education.[12] The vast majority of government spending is composed of transfer payments, defense spending, and interest on the debt. Notably, as discussed in Chapter 1, federal entitlement programs—Social Security, Medicare, Medicaid, and the Affordable Care Act—account for nearly 50 percent of federal spending.[13] Whatever the merits of such programs, they do nothing to increase economic growth.

Moreover, our hypothetical future taxpayers may resist paying the bondholders, especially if they feel that they have neither benefited from the borrowing nor participated in the choice to borrow. Arnold Kling warns that that resistance can create a situation where

> the government will not want to resolve the issue of distributing the cost of the debt. Paying off the debt requires incurring political cost. . . . [T]he political incentive for the government is to go deeper and deeper in debt. This in turn raises the stakes in the political conflict over who will bear the burden

of tax increases and spending reductions. Every year, the debt creates more and more political division and antagonism.[14]

It becomes increasingly difficult for the government to meet its debt obligations, and we can already see some of those political divisions surfacing around issues such as raising the debt ceiling.

There is also an implicit assumption that borrowing, even from ourselves, is what economists call a "frictionless" activity. That is, it has no costs associated with it.

In a frictionless economy, funds are liquid and can flow to the most profitable project or to the person who values the funds most. In reality, however, an economy has limited resources, so the financing of public debt crowds out other investment and expenditure, lowering domestic capital stock, which then lowers future growth. There is, in effect, an opportunity cost to government borrowing. The borrowed money is not available for use by the private sector.

Worse, that opportunity cost is not just a question of substituting a dollar of government spending for a dollar of private spending. Private spending and investment decisions are allocated on the basis of economic forces. People seek the best return on their investments or the best deal on their purchases. Governments allocate much if not most of their spending on the basis of politics. The result is that government spending introduces a host of inefficiencies into the economy, as people and businesses spend time, money, and effort trying to gain government favors or to minimize their share of government costs. Thus, federal borrowing may actually transfer money from wealth-generating activities to unproductive ones, leaving future generations poorer.

The interest payments on the debt, and the way the accumulated public debt affects interest rates, are other sources of friction. Interest must be paid by extracting still more resources from the economy through taxes or additional debt. Interest rates of government bonds, the deposit interest rate, and the lending interest rate can all be affected in different ways as well. Gale and Orszag, for example, report a statistically significant relationship between an increase in government debt of 1 percent of gross domestic product (GDP), sustained for five years, and a rise in the real long-term interest rate by nearly five basis points.[15]

As Buchanan explains, "These are second-order real costs or burdens, over and above that represented by the direct or primary sacrifice of resources actually withdrawn from private usage and subsequently employed by government."[16]

The concept of "owing it to ourselves" may look reasonable on paper, but the reality is not nearly as cost-free as the theory and its proponents suggest.

OK, Debt Is Bad Sometimes, Just Not Now

Even if we can't totally ignore the costs of government borrowing, others argue, current conditions represent a special case when borrowing is justified. Or actually, two different reasons are suggested for why borrowing might be desirable at this time, even if it might not be at other times. The first may be dubbed "necessity," while the other could be considered "favorability."

Those arguing necessity point out that the United States has just gone through one of the deepest economic downturns since the Great Depression, and the recovery has been slow and anemic. Since 2009, economic growth has averaged just 2.25 percent.[17] Unemployment reached 10 percent in October 2009, the highest level since June 1983, and was hovering around 6.2 percent before falling to 5.6 percent in December 2014.[18] That fact may understate the problem since many workers have simply given up looking for work or have accepted part-time jobs.

Keynesian theory suggests that economic downturns may be the result of a decline in consumer spending. It follows then that the way to escape a recession or slow economic growth is to increase consumer spending or "aggregate demand." Unfortunately, the very nature of an economic slowdown prevents the private sector from providing the resources that would boost aggregate demand. Moreover, if consumers anticipate a poor economy in the future, they may decrease spending still further, hoarding their resources and delaying investments. That reaction can create a negative feedback loop, leading to more underconsumption (or oversaving), which then perpetuates lower aggregate demand in the future, and so on.[19] Therefore, it falls to government to break the cycle by increasing demand and consumer spending.

That outcome can be achieved, first, through monetary policy, by reducing interest rates below what would normally be appropriate for a given level of inflation and unemployment. In theory, doing so would decrease saving by lowering the return people can earn on it and would increase spending, since it would be cheaper and easier for people to borrow money. However, in a true liquidity trap, monetary interventions are insufficient to boost behavior. Banks (and individuals) simply don't anticipate a sufficient future return on investment to get them to lend, borrow, or invest.

Keynesians suggest that government must intervene more directly, doing the borrowing and spending itself. Government should run budget deficits when the economy is weak, using the borrowed money to stimulate aggregate demand in society. As the government spending works its way through the economy, consumers will increase their own spending, breaking the cycle and leading to increased economic growth. Once growth has returned, government can cut back on borrowing and spending in order to prevent inflation. In fact, at least some Keynesians hold that in times of strong economic growth, government should run a surplus.[20]

The economic situation following the financial crisis of 2008 would appear to fit the Keynesian definition of a liquidity trap.

In response to the onset of the recession, the Federal Reserve cut the federal funds rate to near zero (approaching the "zero bound") and held it at that lower level for an extended period. Those low interest rates enabled banks to accumulate massive cash reserves because they could borrow most of those funds within the federal funds market at virtually no cost, because the rate was effectively zero. To get a sense of the magnitude of the surge in bank reserves, Federal Reserve data show that in the final months of 2008, the bank reserves in the United States increased by almost a factor of 20, to more than $850 billion. They then went on to almost double from there, as banks continued to stockpile reserves, reaching roughly $1.6 trillion by mid-2011.[21]

At the same time those banks were building up cash reserves that were almost without historical precedent, small businesses stopped taking loans, meaning credit was no longer flowing through the economy. Total borrowing for small businesses plummeted. As Robert Pollin of the University of Massachusetts Amherst notes, for smaller businesses, "total borrowing fell from $546 billion in 2007 to negative $346 billion in 2009—a nearly $900 billion reversal. The non-corporate business sector overall continued to obtain zero net credit over both 2010 and 2011."[22]

Banks were wary of making new loans because they were afraid of losing more money on "risky" investments, and businesses react to the uncertainty in the economic environment by becoming much more risk averse, meaning they were more likely to hold off on expansion plans or take out new loans, regardless of how low the rates were.

At that point, the amount of cash, or liquidity, in the economy was not a key factor in the decisionmaking process for businesses or banks. Credit was already cheap because of the low rates, and banks had an unprecedented amount of cash that was available to loan out. Monetary policy would therefore be ineffective, because it could not further lower the rates, as it was already at or approaching the zero bound. Open-market operations, in which the Fed would try to inject more liquidity by buying up short-term government debt in return for cash, are also ineffective in this scenario. Therefore, since such conventional expansionary monetary policy proves ineffective in a liquidity trap, fiscal stimulus is the preferred policy lever to increase aggregate demand.

Some economists conclude that, although debt may indeed cause problems in the long run, it was necessary to increase deficits (and debt) in the short run in order to "get the economy moving again." As Krugman explains:

> The case for stimulus was that we were suffering from a huge shortfall in overall spending, and that the hit to the economy from the financial crisis and the bursting of the housing bubble was so severe that the Federal Reserve, which normally fights recessions by cutting short-term interest rates, couldn't overcome the slump on its own. The idea, then, was to provide a temporary boost both by having the government directly spend more, and by using tax cuts and public aid to boost family incomes, inducing more private spending.[23]

Many continue, since the economy remains weak, to insist that now is not the time to begin reducing that debt. Someday in the future, we may want to discuss it, but not now.

Although superficially appealing, that Keynesian argument has several flaws.

First, as a practical matter, attempts to stimulate the economy through increased government spending are rarely effective. We can see that in the most recent stimulus. Despite massive borrowing and spending, the recent recovery has been unusually sluggish. With regard to economic growth, it has been the weakest recovery since World War II.[24] And it is the second-worst recovery for job creation.[25]

Why This Failure?

Some Keynesians, such as Krugman, argue that the stimulus was simply too small (or that the effects of the crisis were much worse than originally thought and therefore required a larger stimulus). In reality, however, the stimulus was quite large. Krugman and others tend to focus on the $825 billion stimulus bill that passed in March 2009 (the American Reinvestment and Recovery Act). But that was just one of at least six stimulus proposals under both Presidents Bush and Obama. For example, under President Bush, the Economic Stimulus Act of 2008 gave tax rebates to many Americans, and the Housing and Economic Recovery Act of 2008 sought to bolster the housing market through measures like a first-time homebuyer refundable tax credit for home purchases.

As Robert Samuelson notes, from 2008 to 2013, the federal government ran budget deficits totaling more than $6.2 trillion, roughly 6.4 percent of GDP. Nothing comparable has occurred since World War II. At the same time, the Federal Reserve has added $3.2 trillion to the economy. That's a total injection of close to $9.5 trillion into the economy.[26] How much larger could it have been?

Actually, the failure of Keynesian stimulus to lift us out of recession is far more likely due to flaws in the theory itself. For example, Keynesian theory makes no particular distinction about *how* government money is spent. Indeed, as Keynes once said, the money could be used to dig holes and then fill them back in. Krugman once mused that what this country really needs is an invasion by space aliens. Preparations for an intergalactic war would mean that "this slump would be over in 18 months," he suggested.[27]

In reality, of course, not all government spending is the same. Some government programs actually impede economic growth. At the same time, the realization that government is handing out pots of money generates rent seeking and other unproductive behavior, leading to crony capitalism.

Whatever the Keynesian theory, in practical terms, political considerations have significant effects on the composition of stimulus packages.

Some of those measures are relatively ineffective as economic stimulus, even according to Keynesian theory, and were simply normal budgetary items that were wedged into the bill. Grants to state and local governments (which in many cases did not increase the total amount of spending, because they allowed states to cut back on their own spending) and subsidies for pet industries like green energy and money for school construction are just a few of the examples from the American Reinvestment and Recovery Act.

Moreover, a new study from the St. Louis Fed finds that in the first year of the stimulus, "fewer than one of four stimulus jobs were in the private sector; more than seven of nine jobs in the U.S. economy overall reside in the private sector. Thus, stimulus-funded jobs were heavily tilted toward government."[28] Although those jobs may have had a stimulative effect according to the Keynesian model, they raise other concerns about the sustainability and the size of government, that tendency to be indiscriminate in differentiating between different kinds of spending in the stimulus package both increases the overall cost of the bill and sets a precedent. Some of the more regular provisions were not designed to be temporary and set an elevated spending baseline that can make it more difficult to phase out the spending in later years when the worst effects of the recession have passed.

Part of that effect can be seen in the composition of the American Reinvestment and Recovery Act. Different reports have estimated that only between 50 percent and 64 percent of the stimulus funds were disbursed in the first two years after the bill was passed, with some of those funds not being spent until as many as four years later.[29] However much one may subscribe to Keynesian theory, it is hard to make the case that funds spent in 2012 were an effective stimulus to counteract weak aggregate demand from a recession in 2008. That lag time occurred for two reasons: fiscal policy has an inherent lag in response time as legislation has to wend its way through Congress to passage, and special interests or nonstimulus considerations make their way into the bill and were never really intended to serve as a timely fiscal stimulus anyway. Two years after passage of the stimulus package, more than a third of stimulus spending for contracts, grants, and loans still had yet to be disbursed.[30]

Keynesianism also assumes that economic actors are remarkably myopic. But today's government spending and debt must be paid for at some time in the future. As Harvard's Robert Barro has pointed out, if government runs a deficit, taxpayers will rationally add the value of that deficit to their expected future tax liabilities. In anticipation of having to meet that obligation, they may decrease their expenditures today. To the degree that the decrease in private expenditures offsets the increase in government spending, the net gain to the economy will be zero.[31]

That idea was first expounded by David Ricardo in the 19th century and has become known as Ricardian equivalence.[32] Discussing plans by the British government to pay off its war bonds, Ricardo compared two scenarios for funding the war—one financed it with current taxes, and the other financed it with government bonds—and concluded that the two were equivalent with regards to spending.

That proposition probably overstates the case. People, and even some businesses, are indeed myopic, at least to some degree. It is unlikely that they fully internalize the cost of future taxes.

Still, it would seem silly to deny that a debt as large as ours would have no effect on current spending and investment decisions. At the very least, increased debt today introduces a level of uncertainty that can prevent businesses from investing, expanding, and hiring. We know, for example, that American businesses currently have almost $5 trillion in uninvested assets.[33] Might they not use some of those assets to expand or hire additional workers if they did not fear future taxes?

Beyond the short-term failures of Keynesian stimulus lurks a bigger long-term threat. That is, even if one accepts the need for countercyclical stimulus during times of slow economic growth, fiscal policy is rarely countercyclical during times of positive economic growth. For example, a 2008 paper for the European Commission that looked at euro-area countries from 1980 to 2005 found evidence of procyclical bias in good times, whereas no strong evidence of a cyclical bias is found in bad times.[34] Although in theory governments should follow recessionary spending by cutting back during "boom times," in practice stimulus during recessions is followed by continued fiscal expansion after the recession is over. In other words, spending (and debt) almost always increases regardless of economic conditions (see below).

Debt Is Bad Sometimes, but Not Now (Part 2)

Others argue that current economic conditions, notably low inflation and low interest rates, make for a uniquely favorable opportunity to borrow. Former treasury secretary Larry Summers, for instance, writes, "Governments that enjoy such low borrowing costs can improve their creditworthiness by borrowing more, not less, and investing in improving their future fiscal position, even assuming no positive demand stimulus effects."[35] And Matt Yglesias says, "Under today's interest rate conditions, it's more expensive to pay the bills out of taxes than to just borrow the money, because borrowing is so cheap."[36]

It is true that interest rates are exceptionally low today. Low of course doesn't mean without cost. Interest payments on the federal debt in 2014 totaled $271 billion.[37] To put that in perspective, the sequester has saved less than half that amount, roughly $127 billion through 2014.[38] Still, low interest rates make borrowing attractive if the borrowed funds are then invested in a way that brings a return greater than the interest paid. But as we've repeatedly shown, little government spending brings any return at all.

More important, although interest rates are low today, they are unlikely to remain so into the future when deficit spending and, therefore, borrowing are expected to increase significantly. The Federal Reserve has already signaled its intention to ease its easy money policies and eventually raise interest rates.[39]

Today, the interest rate on three-month T-bills is just 0.02 percent, and 1.98 percent on 10-year notes.[40] According to the Congressional Budget Office (CBO), if interest rates rise to predicted levels—3-month Treasuries to 3.5 percent and 10-year Treasuries to 4.7 percent by 2019— interest payments on the federal debt will reach $492 billion in 2019.[41] As a result, interest payments would be on pace to exceed the cost of all nondefense discretionary spending plus federal civilian retirement programs by 2025, and they will exceed the cost of those programs plus defense—or the entire Social Security program—by 2060.[42]

Debt Is Bad, But We've Licked the Problem

As noted in Chapter 1, budget deficits have been declining since 2011 and were just $483 billion in 2014, their lowest level since 2008, and as little as $469 billion this year. Tax revenues are up, at their highest levels as a percentage of GDP since 2007, and spending, in part thanks to the much-reviled sequester, has fallen to its lowest level, as a percentage of GDP, since 2008.[43]

As a result Krugman and other debt deniers think that either there was never a problem or we have already solved it. Of course, we are still borrowing 20 cents out of every dollar we spend. And more important, that phenomenon is just temporary. According to the CBO's recent report, deficits will start rising as soon as 2016 and by 2024 will approach $1 trillion per year. The CBO also estimates that we will add another $8.77 trillion to the debt through 2024, at which point gross federal debt will be more than $26.5 trillion.[44]

In fact, as Figure 3.1 shows, future debt projections are 2.8 percentage points of GDP higher by 2024 than they were only one year before.[45]

Figure 3.1
Public Debt Projections, 2016–2024

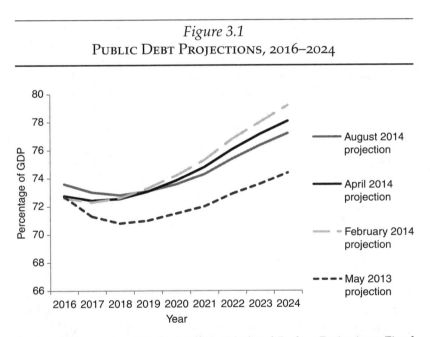

Source: Congressional Budget Office, "Updated Budget Projections: Fiscal Years 2013 to 2023," May 2013; Congressional Budget Office, "The Budget and Economic Outlook: 2014 to 2024," February 2014; Congressional Budget Office, "Updated Budget Projections: 2014 to 2024," April 2014. Congressional Budget Office, "An Update to the Budget and Economic Outlook: 2014 to 2024," August 27, 2014.

The recent deficit reduction carries within it the seeds of its own undoing. That is, having achieved some success in reducing the deficit, Congress will be tempted to increase spending once again.

Indeed, we've already seen movement in that direction. The sequester was a significant factor in slowing the growth of spending since 2012. Yet as part of the 2013 budget agreement, Congress essentially agreed to waive $63 billion in sequester cuts for 2014 and 2015.[46] True, those increases are theoretically offset by undefined cuts to entitlements in 2023 and 2024, but there is more than enough reason to be skeptical about whether those future cuts will ever occur.

Congress also passed, on a bipartisan basis, a massive new farm bill that will cost taxpayers roughly $950 billion over the next 10 years. That amount represents an inflation-adjusted $258 billion increase over the 10-year cost of the last farm bill in 2008, a whopping 37 percent jump in real spending.[47]

In addition, President Obama's FY 2015 budget proposal deliberately eschews what the administration refers to as "austerity," increasing spending by $171 billion over the next 10 years (above the CBO base line).[48] To be fair, the president does project that his budget would result in a gross national debt that is actually $2.2 trillion lower than current projections in 2024, although a still substantial $24.99 trillion.[49] However, the president achieves that debt reduction by relying on extremely rosy projections for economic growth, slowing health care costs, and increased revenues. For example, the president assumes average real GDP growth of 2.7 percent compared with CBO's 2.5 percent projection. The president's budget also anticipates a slightly lower unemployment rate than CBO's, and the president also assumes that a recent slowdown in the growth of health care spending will continue indefinitely.

Several government forecasters, including the CBO and the Medicare system's trustees, remain skeptical (see Chapter 6), but the president relies on that reduction for $402 billion in deficit reduction over 10 years. The president also anticipates more than $1.3 trillion in increased taxes that are included in his budget, but are unlikely to pass Congress in reality. Similarly, the president's budget includes $160 billion in deficit reduction from comprehensive immigration reform.[50] But Republicans in Congress are unlikely to take up the issue this year. Without such rosy scenarios, the president's budget would take gross national debt to a record $26.8 trillion by 2024.[51]

Consider your overweight friend. After years of overeating, he finally cuts back a bit and starts to exercise. As a result, he loses a few pounds. He's still overweight but moving in the right direction. If he decides that his success means he can stop working out and watching what he eats, it won't be long before he's in even worse shape than before he started.

That's a great analogy for the course Washington is taking today.

Besides, We Can't Predict the Future Anyway

Finally, some analysts suggest that concern over long-term debt is premature because the forecasts might simply be wrong. As Matt Yglesias puts it:

> It always strikes me as absurd that it's considered the very height of Washington, D.C., seriousness to pay lots of attention to 75-year budget projections . . . [Go back] in time to the year 1940. Europe is at war, and the United States is clearly casting its lot with the United Kingdom but not directly involved on a military level. People are wondering if tough economic sanctions on Japan will be enough to dissuade it from its brutal efforts to conquer China. There are no antibiotics, jet planes, or television networks. Somebody tells you he has an idea about changing federal health care policy. You ask him, as if it's the most natural question in the world, "What are the implications of your proposal for the federal budget in the year 2012?"[52]

It is true that most budget projections are imprecise. Indeed, most have proved to be wrong over time. But contrary to the implications of the debt deniers, they have not generally overestimated our fiscal obligations; rather they have been too optimistic.

For example, when Medicare was instituted in 1965, government actuaries estimated that the cost of Medicare Part A would be $9 billion by 1990. In actuality, it was seven times higher—$67 billion.[53] Similarly, in 1987, Medicaid's special hospitals subsidy was projected to cost $100 million annually by 1992, just five years later; it actually cost $11 billion, more than 100 times as much.[54] In 1988, when Medicare's home-care benefit was established, the projected cost for 1993 was $4 billion, but the actual cost in 1993 was $10 billion.[55] When the Greenspan Commission "fixed" Social Security in 1983, it predicted that the program's trust fund would be solvent until 2056.[56] The most recent report from the program's trustees warns that the combined trust fund will be exhausted by 2033.[57] And each successive CBO estimate of the cost of the Affordable Care Act has raised its price tag.[58]

Moreover, even if one doubts specific dollar amounts for specific years, there really is little doubt as to direction or trend lines. One can question whether the national debt in 2024 will be $25 trillion or $27 trillion. But does it really make much difference? It will be large, and larger than it is today.

Finally, it hardly seems like sound budgeting to plan on the possibility that you have overestimated your debts. If you are facing enormous credit card bills, you wouldn't want to base your budgetary strategy on the possibility of your winning the lottery someday.

Denial Is Not Just a River in Egypt

When faced with bad news, you have three choices: accept it, ignore it, or deny it. But ignoring or denying something will not change the underlying facts.

A family can continue to pretend that it can live beyond its means, but sooner or later the bills come due. And as a country, we can pretend that we can go on spending and borrowing as if there is no tomorrow. But tomorrow does eventually arrive, and with it the consequences.

4. It's about Entitlements, Stupid

During the 2012 presidential campaign, Mitt Romney was roundly criticized—with some cause—for his remarks about the "47 percent" who do not pay federal income taxes and therefore supposedly were part of the Democratic base.[1] Romney, of course, was factually wrong in implying that the 47 (since fallen to 43.3) percent of Americans who do not pay federal income taxes are some sort of poor underclass. The number includes, for instance, both students who will pay taxes in the future and seniors who paid taxes in the past, as well as others whose circumstances change from year to year. He was perhaps more fundamentally wrong in implying that the poor, whether they pay taxes or not, see themselves as victims and are content to be dependent on government.

And it was just plain silly to say that non–federal taxpayers will uniformly vote for Obama. Although it is true that almost 9 out of 10 nonpayers have incomes below $50,000 per year, the 43.3 percent includes both working poor and middle-class taxpayers with substantial deductions and a large numbers of retirees, who have paid federal taxes in the past, as well as students, who will do so in the future.[2]

Moreover, there is no evidence that most poor people wish to remain permanently dependent on government. Indeed, every survey of those on welfare indicates that they would prefer to be working and aspire to a better life for their children. And some of the nonpaying groups—seniors for example—disproportionately voted for Romney. All in all, Romney's statement was a model of inaccuracy combined with extreme political tone-deafness.

But the dustup over Romney's remarks obscured a larger truth. It's not just who pays taxes that creates a constituency for government spending, although both common sense and academic research suggest that it is easier to increase federal spending if fewer people have to pay for it. "Skin in the game" matters. For example, a study from the nonpartisan Tax Foundation found that "a one percentage point increase in the share of tax filers who are nonpayers is associated with a $10.6 billion per year increase in transfer payments."[3] Given that the percentage of nonpayers has increased by 20 percentage points since 1990 to 41 percent in 2010, the Tax Foundation concluded that the increase over this period is at least partially responsible for $213 billion annually in additional spending.[4] Since 2010 the percentage of nonpayers has increased by another 2.3 percentage points, which could lead to a further $24.38 billion increase in annual transfers.

What really matters is not the number of payers but the number of recipients of government largess. It should be clear that the more people depend on government programs, the harder it becomes to cut those programs. That is not to say that the people on those programs are freeloaders or refuse to take responsibility for their lives. But it does mean that they have a vested interest in maintaining those programs. There is a reason why it is so easy for politicians to demagogue Medicare reform, and why Social Security is the third rail of American politics.

Simply look to what is happening in European countries today. Despite the fact that their welfare states have become unaffordable, any attempt to trim benefits leads to massive resistance. Have we reached that tipping point yet? No, but we may be getting perilously close.

During the 2011 debate over raising the debt ceiling, President Obama noted that the U.S. federal government sends out 70 million checks every month. Unfortunately, that is probably an underestimate. According to the *Washington Post*, the president's estimate included Social Security, veterans' benefits, and spending on nondefense contractors and vendors. But he included neither reimbursements to Medicare providers and vendors nor electronic transfers to the 21 million households receiving food stamps. (Nor did he include most spending by the Defense Department, which has a payroll of 6.4 million active and retired employees and, on average, pays nearly 1 million invoices and 660,000 travel expense claims per month.) The actual number might be closer to 200 million.[5]

A Growing Welfare State

According to the Congressional Budget Office, more than 60 percent of American households receive more in government benefits than they pay in federal taxes.[6] A Tax Foundation study also suggests that, taking into account President Obama's policies, more than 60 percent of Americans are net recipients of government largesse.[7]

As Figure 4.1 shows, in 1966, transfer payments from the federal government made up less than 10 percent of wages and salaries. As recently as 2000, transfer payments amounted to just 21 percent. Today, transfer payments are equivalent to almost 34 percent of all salaries and wages.[8]

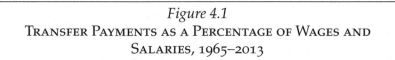

Figure 4.1

TRANSFER PAYMENTS AS A PERCENTAGE OF WAGES AND SALARIES, 1965–2013

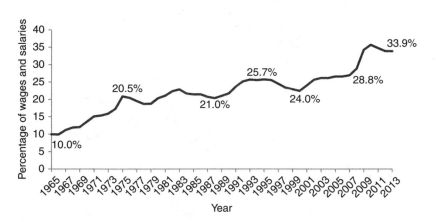

SOURCE: Bureau of Economic Analysis, "National Income and Product Accounts Tables," Table 2.1.

That is not a unique situation brought about by the recent recession and its attendant high levels of unemployment. Growth in the U.S. welfare state has been steady regardless of economic conditions. For example, as Figure 4.1 shows, while transfer payments rose as a percentage of wages during the last major recession from 2001 to

2002, they did not return to previous levels once the recession ended and unemployment declined.[9]

Another way to look at that situation is to consider transfer payments as a proportion of all government spending (Figure 4.2). In 1930, before the Great Depression and Franklin Roosevelt, transfer payments made up roughly 10 percent of total U.S. government spending. By 1969, at the start of Lyndon Johnson's War on Poverty, as well as the enactment of Medicare (and Medicaid), that percentage had almost doubled to 19.7 percent. By 2010, it doubled yet again, reaching almost 41 percent of government spending.[10] That means that the welfare state makes up more than two-fifths of all government spending in the United States.

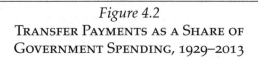

Figure 4.2
TRANSFER PAYMENTS AS A SHARE OF
GOVERNMENT SPENDING, 1929–2013

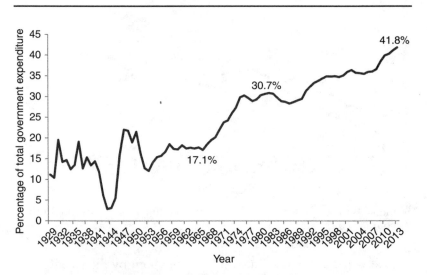

SOURCE: Author's calculations using Bureau of Economic Analysis, "National Income and Product Accounts Tables," Table 2.1; Office of Management and Budget, "Historical Tables," Table 1.1; Federal Reserve Bank of St. Louis, Economic Data, "State and Local Government Total Expenditures" (W079RC1A027NBEA).

Moreover, those income transfers are occurring at higher and higher income levels. In 1979, for example, more than 54 percent of federal transfer payments went to the poorest 20 percent of Americans. But in 2011, just 41 percent did.[11] Thus, transfer payments are increasing, both in absolute terms and as a percentage of federal spending, but they are also increasingly being paid not to the poor but to the middle class. We are no longer simply talking welfare as we have traditionally understood it, but middle-class entitlement programs as well.

That fact is key to dealing with our growing national debt.

How Government Spends Our Money

Figure 4.3 shows how the federal government actually spends its money. Politicians like to pretend that you can deal with the debt

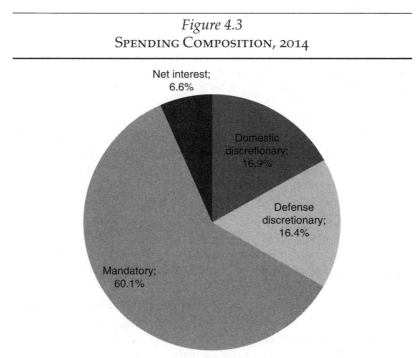

Figure 4.3
Spending Composition, 2014

2014 Expenditures

Source: Congressional Budget Office, "An Update to the Budget and Economic Outlook: 2014 to 2024," August 27, 2014.

crisis by eliminating "fraud, waste, and abuse" in the federal budget, and certainly there is plenty of that. But you simply cannot balance the budget by cutting the usual suspects. Foreign aid amounts to less than 1 percent of federal spending. Federal subsidies to Planned Parenthood and the Corporation for Public Broadcasting amount to a combined 0.0002 percent.

In fact, all domestic discretionary spending—everything from the Department of Education and the Federal Bureau of Investigation, to National Aeronautics and Space Administration and the Food and Drug Administration—accounts for just 16.9 percent of all federal spending.[12] Of course, that doesn't mean that discretionary spending can't or shouldn't be cut. After all, since 2000, nondefense discretionary spending has increased by 80 percent.[13] Still, we are not going to solve our spending problem just on the discretionary side of the budget.

Moreover, the sequester and recent budgets have significantly reduced discretionary spending both as a share of the economy and as a share of the deficit. Domestic discretionary spending will amount to just 3.28 percent of gross domestic product (GDP) in 2015 and will fall to just 2.48 percent by 2024. That will be the lowest level in more than 50 years.

As described previously, defense discretionary spending, which constitutes roughly 16.4 percent of federal spending, can and should be cut as well. Another 6.6 cents out every dollar that the federal government spends is for interest on our current federal debt. That area of government, unfortunately, cannot be reduced by legislative action, at least in the short term.

Everything else falls under the broad heading of entitlement, or mandatory, spending, which accounts for 60.1 percent of federal spending. In particular, three entitlement programs—Social Security, Medicare, and Medicaid—account for almost 50 cents of every dollar that the federal government spends.[14]

In simple dollar terms, in 2015 we will spend $887 billion on Social Security this year and $620 billion on Medicare, while the federal government's portion of Medicaid spending will amount to $328 billion. That's a total of $1.836 trillion out of a $3.75 trillion federal budget. That's roughly as much (on an inflation-adjusted basis) as the entire federal government spent in 1982. And it is more than the entire GDP of such countries as Australia, Mexico, Poland, Spain, Sweden, Switzerland, and many others.[15]

That factor represents an ongoing change in the way that the federal government spends money. As Figure 4.4 shows, entitlement spending has been rising as a share of the federal budget since the 1960s, while both domestic and defense discretionary spending have been declining.

Figure 4.4
Distribution of Federal Outlays, 1962–2013

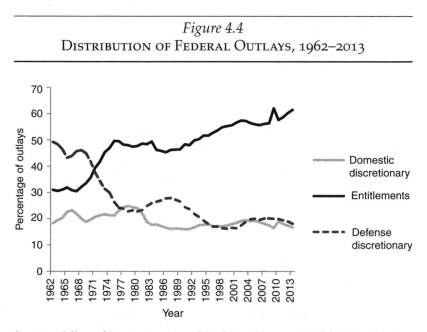

SOURCE: Office of Management and Budget, "Historical Tables," Table 8.3.

Actually, It's the Entitlement State

The term "entitlement" itself is the subject of much confusion. For example, many seniors object to calling Social Security and Medicare entitlements, claiming that the term brands those programs as a form of welfare, when in fact seniors have paid taxes into those programs. However, even setting aside the issue of whether those complaints properly characterize payroll taxes, they misunderstand the meaning of entitlement.

Entitlement is actually a legal and budgetary term that describes a program not subject to annual appropriation. Congress does not vote on their budgets every year. Rather, the programs spend whatever is necessary to provide statutory benefits under broad categories of eligibility. In other words, if you have reached retirement age and are otherwise eligible, you receive Social Security benefits. Whatever is necessary to provide those benefits to all eligible recipients will be spent. In fact, that is what differentiates entitlement spending from discretionary spending. There is no discretion about how much to spend. It's pretty much on autopilot.

By that definition, Social Security and Medicare, as well as programs like farm price supports, are entitlements, but—perhaps ironically—most traditional welfare programs such as Temporary Assistance to Needy Families are not.

Returning to Figure 4.3, it should be obvious that no matter how deep we cut into defense and domestic discretionary spending, we will not solve our debt problems in that way. Of course, that is not an argument against cutting defense or discretionary spending. Congress should cut wherever possible. But ultimately, any serious plan to balance the budget long term and to reduce the size and cost of government must address Social Security, Medicare, and Medicaid.

And as much of federal spending as we devote to those three programs today, they are going to take even more in the future. Thus, entitlements will gradually squeeze out everything else in the budget.

Consider this: By 2035, Medicare, Medicaid, and Social Security will consume roughly 13.9 percent of GDP, while interest on the federal debt will amount to another 4.3 percent of GDP.[16] If one assumes that revenues return to and stay at their traditional 17.3 percent of GDP, then those three entitlement programs plus interest will consume all federal revenues. Not a single dime would be available for any other program of government, from national defense to welfare.

The Affordable Care Act contributes to this entitlement burden, since it both expands Medicaid and adds its own entitlement in the form of subsidies for the purchase of insurance. By 2024, it will contribute half a percentage point of GDP in government spending and consume 3 percent of federal spending.[17]

We've Been Warned

It is not as though there has been no warning about entitlement growth. As far back as 1995, the Bipartisan Commission on Entitlement and Tax Reform was pointing out: "If we do not plan for the future, entitlement spending promises will exceed federal resources in the next century. The current trend is unsustainable." The commissioners went on to warn, "If we fail to act, we have made a choice that threatens the economic future of our children and the nation."[18] Four years later, the National Bipartisan Commission on the Future of Medicare, while unable to reach a consensus on how to reform the program, concluded that it was unsustainable in its present form.[19] Likewise, President Clinton's Advisory Council on Social Security agreed that Social Security, as currently structured, could not meet its future obligations.[20]

If anything, those warnings—over many years and across political and ideological differences—have understated the threat to future generations. But so far, both political parties have sought partisan political advantage rather than dealing with the looming threat. Democrats demagogued President Bush's attempts to allow younger workers to privately invest a portion of their Social Security taxes and continue to attack any Republican who raises the issue.[21] Republicans criticized Democrats for daring to make cuts, however tentative, in Medicare as part of their health care reform effort.[22]

Indeed, Nicholas Eberstadt notes that entitlement spending has actually grown faster under Republican presidents than under Democrats, on average 8 percent faster on a year-over-year basis.[23] Nor should we forget that it was George W. Bush who pushed through Medicare's prescription drug benefit, the largest expansion of entitlements since Lyndon Johnson created Medicare and Medicaid. Entitlement spending is not a partisan issue.

The reason why previous warnings about entitlements have gone unheeded is easy to see. Fully 86 percent of all Americans age 65 and older receive Social Security.[24] Moreover, 5.7 million seniors also receive Medicaid to cover their long-term care (i.e., nursing home) expenses.[25] More than a tenth of the elderly receive benefits from all three programs.

They depend on those benefits for a substantial portion of their retirement income. For example, 46 percent of elderly married couples and 65.5 percent of unmarried persons over 65 receive more than half or more of their income from Social Security. [26] Almost 42 percent of unmarried seniors rely on Social Security for at least 90 percent of their income, and nearly 19 percent of elderly married couples do.[27] Medicare pays for 54 percent of health care spending by seniors.[28] And although Medicaid is generally thought of as a program for the poor, in reality 23 percent of Medicaid spending actually goes to seniors, primarily to pay for long-term care.[29] Medicaid pays for 41 percent of all long-term care in this country.[30]

Any entitlement reform, therefore, must take into account the dependence that we've already built up among seniors. That is both practical—it's difficult and unfair to change the rules for seniors in the middle of the game—and political.

Seniors are a powerful voting bloc. In the 2012 elections, voters over age 65 made up more than 22 percent of the registered voters who reported they voted in the elections. Those under age 30 composed just 15.4 percent.[31] And of course, those under 18 and generations yet unborn do not vote at all. That fact makes for a powerful incentive for Congress to provide benefits to seniors, while passing the bill on to young people and future generations.

The Clock Is Ticking

Simply put, there is no way to reduce the growth in government spending and debt without reforming entitlements.

The following chapters take a more detailed look at each of those programs and offer some options for reform. None of those reforms will be politically easy. If they were, they would have already been implemented. But the longer we put off action, the more difficult and painful it will be to implement any changes.

5. Social Security: Facing Up to Ponzi

During the 2012 Republican presidential primaries, Texas governor Rick Perry came under fire for having written that Social Security is "set up like an illegal Ponzi scheme."[1] He explicitly compared Social Security's financing with the type of illegal scheme "that sent Bernie Madoff to prison," explaining that, like a Ponzi scheme, "deceptive accounting has hoodwinked the American people into thinking that Social Security is a retirement system and financially sound when clearly it is not."[2]

Perry's statement was roundly denounced by other Republican candidates, especially the eventual Republican nominee, former Massachusetts governor Mitt Romney, as well as many Social Security advocates and large portions of the media.

Yet Social Security has many structural characteristics that resemble those of the classic Ponzi or pyramid scheme. For example, like a Ponzi scheme, Social Security does not actually save or invest any of a participant's payments. When a worker pays taxes into the system, that money is used to pay current beneficiaries. Therefore, participants receive payments, not from returns on their own investments but directly from inflows from subsequent participants.

As a result, Social Security was able to pay early participants a windfall return on the money that they paid in taxes.[3] But as demographic changes result in fewer workers paying into the program and more recipients taking benefits out, the return to subsequent generations grows steadily worse. Today's young workers will receive a rate of return far lower than what they could receive from private markets.

Indeed, both opponents and supporters of Social Security have long noted the program's pyramid-like structure. Milton Friedman called Social Security "the biggest Ponzi scheme on earth."[4] So did his fellow Nobel laureate Paul Samuelson, who famously referred to Social Security as "a Ponzi scheme that works."[5] That sentiment was echoed by Paul Krugman, who has written of Social Security's

"Ponzi game aspect, in which each generation takes more out than it put in."[6]

Of course, there is one crucial distinction between Social Security and a Ponzi scheme. Once Ponzi was unable to talk enough people into investing with him, his scheme collapsed. People participate in Social Security because the government makes them. And if the Social Security system begins to run short of people paying into the system, as it is now, it can force those people to pay more.

Yet Congress's ability to preserve Social Security through higher taxes and lower benefits should not distract from the fundamental fact that Social Security is unable to pay the promised level of benefits with current levels of revenue. It faces unfunded future liabilities in excess of $24.9 trillion and will be the second-largest contributor to this country's long-term debt, after Medicare.

The Growth of Social Security

The Social Security Act was signed into law by President Franklin Delano Roosevelt on August 14, 1935. The United States was actually a latecomer to the idea of a government-provided old-age pension program, first introduced by Chancellor Otto von Bismarck in Germany in 1889. In fact, by the time that Roosevelt signed the Social Security Act, 35 countries, mostly in Europe and Latin America, had already established such programs.

The Social Security Act imposed a 1 percent tax on employees' wages to be matched by a 1 percent tax on employers, starting in 1937. The amount of wages subject to the tax was capped at $3,000, making the maximum tax $60 ($30 by the employee and $30 by the employer).[7] Benefits were paid beginning in 1940.

Originally, the Social Security program was quite modest. Not only were both the taxes and benefits relatively low, but the program did not apply to agricultural workers, domestic servants, casual laborers, seamen, government workers, and employees of any non-profit organization, including educational, religious, and scientific organizations. Those other categories of workers were gradually included in the years since, most added by President Harry Truman in 1952, with government workers being brought into the system only in 1984.

Social Security also originally provided only retirement benefits. Truman added survivors benefits in 1952, and disability benefits were added to the program in 1956. Over the same period, the level of retirement benefits, and the taxes necessary to pay for them, increased dramatically.

However, if the period between Social Security's birth and the mid-1970s was marked by an almost uninterrupted expansion of the program, in both the scope of coverage and benefits provided, as well as the level of the benefits themselves, storm clouds were on the horizon. By the mid-1970s, it was becoming apparent that Social Security could not continue to finance all the benefits it had promised. In 1975, for the first time since 1959, Social Security ran a deficit, spending more on benefits than it brought in through taxes. The same thing happened in 1976 and 1977. Operating deficits were projected to continue in subsequent years, and reserves would be exhausted by the early 1980s. Congress and President Jimmy Carter responded with the largest tax increase in American history (until that time). In signing the changes, Carter announced, "From 1980 through 2030, the Social Security system will be sound."[8]

He was wrong. By 1983, Social Security was again teetering on the edge of insolvency. Projections showed that Social Security faced a deficit of $150 billion to $200 billion between 1983 and 1989, with a 75-year shortfall of more than $1.6 trillion. Indeed, by some estimates, Social Security would be unable to pay benefits by July 1983.

A commission had been established in 1982, chaired by Alan Greenspan and including representatives from Congress, business, and labor, to propose long-term reforms to Social Security. By 1983, facing the possibility that checks might actually be delayed for millions of retirees, the committee agreed to a set of recommendations combining modest benefit restraint and a large increase in the payroll tax.[9] Pushed by both President Reagan and House Speaker Tip O'Neill, Congress quickly passed those reforms, as well as a gradual increase in the retirement age from 65 to 67 by 2027.

Once again, program supporters pronounced the program fiscally sound, predicting solvency until at least 2062. Once again, they were wrong.

By the mid-1990s, it was apparent that Social Security's finances were once more deteriorating rapidly. President Bill Clinton launched a nationwide campaign to consider proposals that would "Save Social Security First." The Clinton administration actively considered proposals for personal accounts and even established a Treasury Department task force to look into how a personal account system could be implemented. Unfortunately, the Lewinsky scandal and the threat of impeachment arose. In the end, nothing was done to reform the program, and Social Security's finances grew steadily worse.

George W. Bush was the next president to consider Social Security reform. His first effort, which included a bipartisan commission headed by Democratic Senator Daniel Patrick Moynihan, was derailed by the terrorist attack on 9/11. Bush launched a second, more sustained campaign for reform during his second term. Unfortunately, by that time, the president's credibility had been greatly diminished by the war in Iraq, the response to Hurricane Katrina, and other failures. In the face of a furious opposition campaign led by AARP and labor unions, the reform effort collapsed.

President Obama has offered only the most tepid support for Social Security reform. He has occasionally voiced support for some restraint in the growth of future benefits, such as changing the formula for calculating cost-of-living adjustments.[10] More recently, he has backed away from even that idea.[11]

Social Security's problems, however, have not gone away.

Social Security Basics

Social Security today is the largest program operated by the federal government. Indeed, it is the largest government program in the world, providing more than $812 billion in benefits to almost 58 million recipients in 2013.[12] Social Security accounts for more than 20 percent of all federal spending, more than the amount that the federal government will spend on all other entitlement programs, except Medicare, combined.

Social Security provides a variety of benefits, the major ones being retirement benefits, including spousal benefits, disability, and survivors benefits. Indeed, the full name of the program that we call Social Security is actually the Old-Age, Survivors, and Disability Insurance Program. Although interrelated, the various aspects of Social Security are technically funded (at least in part) by distinct and dedicated portions of the Social Security payroll tax, and actually have separate trust funds.

Retirement benefits: Social Security has become the primary source of retirement income for most Americans. Approximately 35 percent of all income for individuals age 65 or older comes from Social Security benefits.[13] Almost three-quarters of elderly Americans have no private pension, and almost half have no income from assets.[14]

In 2013, Social Security paid out almost $529 billion in retirement benefits to 40.8 million American retirees and auxiliaries. That amount represented more than 65 percent of the program's expenditures.

In determining an individual's Social Security retirement benefits, the Social Security Administration (SSA) first calculates his or her Average Indexed Monthly Earnings (AIME). All earnings on which the person has paid Social Security taxes between 1968 and the year in which he or she reaches age 60 are indexed to account for past inflation and real wage growth. The indexing formula is based on the ratio of the average national wage in the year the individual turns 60 to the year to be indexed. Wages earned after age 60 are not indexed but are left in nominal dollars. The SSA then selects the 35 years in which wages are highest. The wages for those years are totaled and divided by 420 months. The result is the AIME.[15]

From that amount, a progressive formula is used to determine the person's Primary Insurance Amount (PIA). For people reaching the full retirement age of 66 in 2015, that formula was 90 percent of the first $826 of the AIME, plus 32 percent of the next $4,980 of the AIME, plus 15 percent of the remaining AIME.[16]

In the case of early or late retirement, benefits are adjusted accordingly. For example, if a worker retires at age 62 (the earliest allowable age under Social Security) the worker's benefits will be *permanently* reduced to 80 percent of his or her PIA. If the worker delays retirement until age 67, his benefit will be increased to 108 percent of PIA.[17]

Spousal benefits: A spouse who has not worked long enough to be eligible for her own benefits will, at age 62, receive benefits equal to 50 percent of the worker's PIA.[18]

Survivors benefits: Social Security also provides benefits to surviving spouses and to children under the age of 18. In 2013, Social Security paid out more than $112 billion in survivors benefits to

6.2 million Americans. That amount represented almost 14 percent of Social Security's total expenditures.[19]

If a worker dies, a surviving spouse over age 60 receives benefits equal to 100 percent of the worker's PIA. If the widowed spouse is under age 60, she is eligible for benefits equal to 75 percent of the PIA if she is caring for children under age 16. Minor children of a deceased worker are also eligible for survivors benefits equal to 75 percent of the PIA. However, a family's total benefits are capped at between 150 percent and 188 percent of the PIA, according to a mildly progressive formula.[20]

Disability benefits: Finally, Social Security also provides benefits to disabled workers, defined as those workers with a physical or mental impairment that prevents them from performing "substantial" work for at least a year. Generally, earnings of $1,040 or more per month are considered substantial work. Further, the disability must generally be considered permanent.

In 2013, Social Security paid out $140 billion in disability benefits to 10.98 million disabled workers and their dependents, roughly 17.2 percent of the program's expenditures.[21]

Disability benefits are generally equal to the individual's PIA, computed as though he or she were age 62 at the time of disablement. If the person is receiving workers compensation or other types of government disability benefits, the Social Security disability payment may be reduced.[22]

The Looming Crisis

Social Security is a *pay-as-you-go* (PAYGO) program, in which Social Security taxes are used to immediately pay benefits for current retirees. It is not a *funded* plan, where contributions are accumulated and invested in financial assets and liquidated and converted into a pension at retirement. Rather, it is a simple wealth transfer from current workers to current retirees.

Table 5.1 shows a basic model of overlapping generations, where people are born in every time period, live for two periods (the first as workers, the second as retirees), and finally die. As time passes, older generations are replaced by younger generations. The columns represent successive time periods, and the rows represent successive generations. Each generation is labeled by the period of its birth, so that Generation 1 is born in Period 1, and so on. In each period, two generations overlap, with younger workers coexisting with older retirees.

In Table 5.1, a PAYGO pension system provides a start-up bonus to Generation 0 retirees by taking contributions from Generation 1 workers to pay out benefits to those already retired. The PAYGO program provides initial (Generation 0) retirees a windfall because they never paid taxes into the system. Subsequent generations both pay taxes and receive benefits. There is no direct relationship between taxes paid and benefits received.[23]

Table 5.1
A PAYGO Social Security System

	Period 1	**Period 2**	**Period 3**	**Period 4**
Generation 0	Retired benefits	Dead	Dead	Dead
Generation 1	↑ Working ↑ contributions	Retired benefits	Dead	Dead
Generation 2	Unborn	↑ Working ↑ contributions	Retired benefits	Dead
Generation 3	Unborn	Unborn	↑ Working ↑ contributions	Retired benefits
Generation 4	Unborn	Unborn	Unborn	↑ Working ↑ contributions

Source: Thomas F. Siems, "Reengineering Social Security for the New Economy," Cato Institute Project on Social Security Privatization, SSP no. 22, January 23, 2001.

As long as the wage base supporting Social Security grows faster than the number of recipients, the program can continue to pay higher benefits to those recipients. But the growth in the labor force has slowed dramatically. In 1950, for example, there were 16 workers paying taxes into the system for every retiree receiving benefits from the program. However, Americans have been living longer and having fewer babies. As a result, there are now just 2.8 workers per beneficiary, and by 2030 there will be only 2.2 (see Figure 5.1).[24] And real wage growth (especially in wages below the payroll tax cap) has not been nearly fast enough to offset that demographic shift.

Figure 5.1
WORKER-TO-BENEFICIARY RATIO, 1945–2090

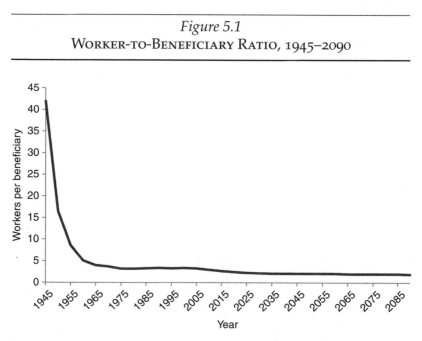

SOURCE: *The 2014 Annual Report of the Board of Trustees of the Federal Old-Age and Survivors Insurance and Federal Disability Insurance Trust Funds* (Washington: Government Printing Office, July 28, 2014).

In 2013, Social Security spent $99.1 billion more on benefits than it took in through taxes.[25] In part, that shortfall was the result of the temporary reduction in payroll taxes passed in 2011, and extended for an additional year in 2012, before being allowed to expire on January 1, 2013, as part of the deal to avert the fiscal cliff. However, even though the payroll tax has returned to its full 12.4 percent rate, Social Security still received almost $31 billion in general revenue reimbursements for the payroll tax reduction, which drove up the cash-flow shortfall in 2013. Although things will improve in 2014 as the effects of the temporary payroll tax reduction finally dissipate, things only get worse after that (Figure 5.2).[26]

Figure 5.2
CASH-FLOW DEFICIT, 2014–2024

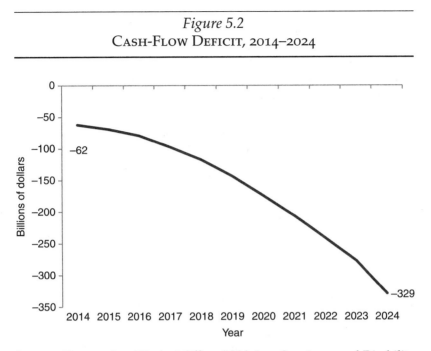

SOURCE: Congressional Budget Office, "Old-Age, Survivors, and Disability Insurance Trust Funds—CBO's April 2014, Baseline," April 14, 2014.

In theory, of course, Social Security is supposed to continue paying benefits by drawing on the Social Security Trust Fund until 2033, after which the trust fund will be exhausted.[27] At that point, by law, Social Security benefits will have to be cut by approximately 23 percent.[28]

However, in reality, the Social Security Trust Fund is not an asset that can be used to pay benefits. As the Clinton administration's fiscal year 2000 budget explained it:

> These [Trust Fund] balances are available to finance future benefit payments and other Trust Fund expenditures—but only in a bookkeeping sense. . . . They do not consist of real economic assets that can be drawn down in the future to fund benefits. Instead, they are claims on the Treasury that, when redeemed, will have to be financed by raising taxes, borrowing from the public, or reducing benefits or other

> expenditures. The existence of large Trust Fund balances, therefore, does not, by itself, have any impact on the Government's ability to pay benefits.[29]

Even if Congress can find a way to redeem the bonds, the trust fund surplus will be completely exhausted by 2033.[30] At that point, Social Security will have to rely solely on revenue from the payroll tax— but that revenue will not be sufficient to pay all promised benefits. Overall, Social Security faces unfunded liabilities of $24.9 trillion ($27.63 trillion if the cost of redeeming the trust fund is included).[31] Clearly, Social Security is not sustainable in its current form. Consequently, Congress will again be forced to resort to raising taxes, cutting benefits, or both in order to enable the program to stumble along.

In fact, the benefit estimate mailed to workers annually by the SSA contains this disclaimer:

> Your estimated benefits are based on current law. Congress has made changes to the law in the past and can do so at any time. The law governing benefit amounts may change because, by 2033, the payroll taxes collected will be enough to pay only about 77 percent of scheduled benefits."[32]

In short, no matter what the official promise of your benefits, Social Security will not really be able to pay all of them.

Other Issues with Social Security

Social Security taxes are already so high, relative to benefits, that Social Security has quite simply become a bad deal for younger workers, providing a poor, below-market rate of return. That poor rate of return means that many young workers' retirement benefits are far lower than if they had been able to invest those funds privately.

In addition, Social Security taxes displace private savings options, resulting in a large net loss of national savings, reducing capital investment, wages, national income, and economic growth. Moreover, by increasing the cost of hiring workers, the payroll tax substantially reduces wages, employment, and economic growth as well.

After all the economic analysis, however, perhaps the single most important reason for transforming Social Security into a system of individual accounts is that it would give American workers true ownership of and control over their retirement benefits.

Many Americans believe that Social Security is an "earned right." That is, because they have paid Social Security taxes, they are entitled to receive Social Security benefits. The government encourages that belief by referring to Social Security taxes as "contributions," as in FICA (Federal Insurance Contributions Act). However, in the case of *Flemming v. Nestor*, the U.S. Supreme Court ruled that workers have no legally binding contractual or property right to their Social Security benefits, and those benefits can be changed, cut, or even taken away at any time.

As the Court stated, "To engraft upon Social Security a concept of 'accrued property rights' would deprive it of the flexibility and boldness in adjustment to ever changing conditions which it demands."[33] That decision built on a previous case, *Helvering v. Davis*, in which the Court had ruled that Social Security is not a contributory insurance program, stating that "the proceeds of both the employer and employee taxes are to be paid into the Treasury like any other internal revenue generally, and are not earmarked in any way."[34]

In effect, Social Security turns older Americans into supplicants, dependent on the political process for their retirement benefits. If they work hard, play by the rules, and pay Social Security taxes their entire lives, they earn the privilege of going hat in hand to the government and hoping that politicians decide to give them some money for retirement.

Options for Reform

And there are really few options for dealing with the problem. That is not an opinion shared only by supporters of individual accounts. As former president Bill Clinton pointed out, the only ways to keep Social Security solvent are to

- raise taxes,
- cut benefits,
- get a higher rate of return through private capital investment.[35]

Certainly, throughout its history, Social Security taxes have been raised frequently to keep the system financially viable. The initial Social Security tax was 2 percent (split between the employer and employee), capped at $3,000 of earnings. That made for a maximum tax of $60. Since then, as Figure 5.3 shows, the payroll tax rate and the ceiling at which wages are subject to the tax have been raised a combined total of 67 times. Today, the tax is 12.4 percent, capped at $118,500, for a maximum tax of $14,694.[36] Even adjusting for inflation, that rate represents more than an 800 percent increase.

Figure 5.3
PAYROLL TAX RATE AND TAXABLE MAXIMUM INCREASES, 1938–2015

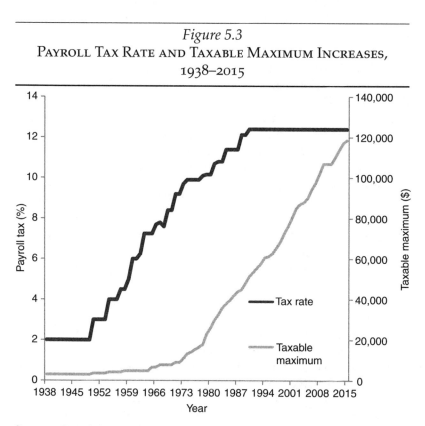

SOURCE: Social Security Administration, "Contribution and Benefit Base," http://www.ssa.gov/oact/cola/cbb.html.

On the other hand, Congress can reduce Social Security benefits. Restoring the program to solvency would require at least a 23 percent reduction in benefits. Suggested changes include further raising the retirement age, trimming cost-of-living adjustments, means testing, or changing the wage price indexing formula.

Congress has occasionally reduced benefits in the past. For example, in 1993, the Social Security retirement age was increased for workers age 45 and younger at the time.[37] Since the amount of payments a recipient will receive over a lifetime depends in part on how long they collect benefits, delaying the age at which they begin to receive those benefits effectively reduces the total amount of those benefits. Thus, although it is technically true that, as the Social Security Administration claims, "it has never missed a payment," it has paid less than originally promised.

Obviously, there are better and worse ways to make those changes. But as we saw earlier, most younger workers will receive returns far below those provided by private investment. Some will actually receive less in benefits than they pay into the system, a negative return. Both tax hikes and benefit reductions further reduce the return that workers can expect on their contributions (taxes).

A Better Reform: Personal Accounts

In the end, raising taxes or cutting benefits are little more than Band-Aids. A permanent fix will require changing Social Security from the PAYGO model that so resembles a Ponzi scheme to a system where at least some of an individual's Social Security taxes are saved for a person's retirement and invested in real assets.

Table 5.2 shows what that change would mean. Unlike the current Social Security system, each working generation's contributions would actually be saved and would accumulate as time passes. That accumulation, including the returns earned through real investment, would then be used to pay that generation's benefits when they retire. Under a funded system, there would be no transfer from current workers to current retirees. Each generation would pay for its own retirement.[38]

Table 5.2
A FUNDED SOCIAL SECURITY SYSTEM

Generation	Period 1	Period 2	Period 3	Period 4
0		Dead	Dead	Dead
1	Working → contributions	Retired benefits	Dead	Dead
2	Unborn	Working → contributions	Retired benefits	Dead
3	Unborn	Unborn	Working → contributions	Retired benefits
4	Unborn	Unborn	Unborn	Working → contributions

SOURCE: Thomas F. Siems, "Reengineering Social Security for the New Economy," Cato Institute Project on Social Security Privatization, SSP no. 22, January 23, 2001.

In this system, there is a direct link between contributions and benefits. Workers in each generation receive benefits equal to their contribution plus the returns their investments earn. And because real investment takes place, and the rate of return on capital investment can be expected to exceed the growth in wages, workers can expect to receive higher returns than under the current system.

Although from a strictly economic viewpoint it makes no difference whether investment under such a funded system is made by the government directly or through personal accounts, one need look no further than the Troubled Asset Relief Program or the auto industry bailout to see reasons for concern with government investment. If the goal is to move away from a Ponzi-style PAYGO system to a program based on savings and investment, a much better approach is to allow younger workers to save at least a portion of their payroll taxes through individual accounts.[39]

Moving to a system of individual accounts would allow workers to take advantage of the potentially higher returns available from capital investment. In a dynamically efficient economy, the return to capital will exceed the rate of return to labor and therefore will be higher than the benefits that Social Security can afford to pay.

In the United States, the return on capital has generally run about 2.5 percentage points higher than the return on labor.[40]

True, capital markets are both risky and volatile. But private capital investment remains remarkably safe over the long term. Despite recent declines in the stock market, a worker who had invested over the past 40 years would have still earned an average yearly return of 6.85 percent investing in the S&P 500, 3.46 percent from corporate bonds, and 2.44 percent from government bonds.[41]

For example, a 2012 Cato Institute study found that if workers retiring in 2011, near the nadir of the stock market's recession-era decline, had been allowed to invest the employee half of the Social Security payroll tax over their working lifetime, they would retire with *more* income than if they relied on Social Security.[42] Indeed, even in the worst-case scenario, a low-wage worker who invested entirely in bonds, the benefits from private investment would equal those from traditional Social Security.[43] Although that type by analysis has limits and caveats, it clearly shows that the argument that private investment is too risky compared with Social Security does not hold up.

Low-income workers would be among the biggest winners under a system of privately invested individual accounts. Private investment would pay low-income workers significantly higher benefits than Social Security could pay. And that does not take into account the fact that blacks, other minorities, and the poor have below-average life expectancies. As a result, they tend to live fewer years in retirement and collect less in Social Security benefits than do whites.[44] In a system of individual accounts, by contrast, they would each retain control over the funds paid in and could pay themselves higher benefits over their fewer retirement years or could leave more to their children or other heirs.

The higher returns and benefits of a private, invested system would be most important to low-income families, as they most need the extra funds. The funds saved in the individual retirement accounts, which could be left to the children of the poor, would also greatly help families break out of the cycle of poverty. Similarly, the improved economic growth, higher wages, and increased jobs that would result from an investment-based Social Security system would be most important to the poor. Without reform, low-income workers will be hurt the most by the higher taxes or reduced benefits that will be necessary if we continue on our current course.

In addition, with average- and low-wage workers accumulating large sums in their own investment accounts, the distribution of wealth throughout society would become far broader than it is today.

Recently, much discussion has taken place in this country about wealth inequality. Thomas Piketty's new book, *Capital in the Twenty-First Century*, for example, argues that the accumulation of capital by the wealthy in modern capitalist economies is "potentially threatening to democratic societies and to the values of social justice on which they are based."[45]

But no policy proposed in recent years would do more to expand capital ownership than allowing younger workers to invest a portion of their Social Security taxes through personal accounts. It would enable even the lowest-paid American worker to benefit from capital investment.

In Chile, for example, workers, through their pension accounts, own assets equal to approximately 60 percent of the country's gross domestic product. As José Piñera, the architect of Chile's successful pension reform, points out, personal accounts "transform every worker into an owner of capital."[46] Moreover, Jagadeesh Gokhale, formerly my colleague at the Cato Institute and now with the Wharton Public Policy Initiative, has demonstrated that, because personal accounts would be inheritable, privatizing Social Security would significantly reduce inequality across generations.[47]

Shifting to a private system, with hundreds of billions of dollars invested in individual accounts each year, would also produce a large net increase in national savings, depending on how the government financed the transition. That increase in savings would increase national investment, productivity, wages, jobs, and economic growth.[48] Replacing the payroll tax with private retirement contributions would also improve economic growth because the required contributions would be lower and would be viewed as part of a worker's direct compensation, stimulating more employment and output.

As far as federal spending goes, it should be noted, however, that although moving to a system of individual accounts will save money in the long run, it will increase deficits in the short term. The reason is, to the degree that workers choose the individual account option, payroll tax revenues are redirected from the payment of current benefits to being saved in the accounts.

It is important to remember though that the financing of that transition is a one-time event that actually serves to reduce the government's future liabilities.[49] The transition moves the program's shortfalls forward in time, but—depending on the transition's ultimate design—it does not increase the amount of spending necessary. In effect, it is a case of "pay a little now or pay a lot later."

The Necessity for Reform

The failure of President George W. Bush's bungled 2005 campaign for personal accounts is widely believed to have taken that idea off the table for the foreseeable future. None of the recent deficit commissions included personal accounts in their recommendations.

But Social Security's problems have not gone away, and the more traditional solutions (raising taxes or cutting benefits) come with their own political difficulties. Several reform-minded representatives and senators were elected in 2010 and 2012. As a result, there may be more interest in the next Congress.

In the end, however, the question of Social Security reform is one not of politics but of math. Social Security simply cannot pay the promised level of future benefits with the amount of revenue that the system will be bringing in. Sooner or later the Ponzi scheme will collapse. The only thing left to ask, therefore, is whether our political leaders will have the courage to act before it does.

6. Medicare: The 800–Pound Gorilla

For all the problems that Social Security is facing, that program is really the low-hanging fruit of the entitlement debate. Medicare is a bigger problem and one much harder to fix.

This year alone, Medicare cost taxpayers more than $530 billion, roughly 15 percent of the entire federal budget.[1] That figure makes Medicare the second-largest federal government program, behind Social Security. Health care costs in general, and spending on Medicare, have grown more slowly in recent years. To some extent, that slowdown has slightly improved the fiscal outlook of the program, but much of this slowdown is due to the lingering effects of the recession, and spending is projected to return to a higher rate of growth in the coming years. One study by David Dranove and colleagues at the Kellogg School of Management estimates that the economic effects of the recession account for 70 percent of the slowdown in health-spending growth.[2] Another study by the Kaiser Family Foundation found that the recession and broader economic effects accounted for 77 percent of the slowdown.[3] In both of those studies, the one-off effects of the recession were responsible for the majority of the slowdown, and the growth in health care costs is expected to revert to higher levels in the future. According to the Congressional Budget Office (CBO), Medicare spending will increase at a rate of almost 6 percent per year, reaching at least $1 trillion annually by 2023.[4]

That escalating cost will add heavily to America's debt burden. The program's trustees warn that Medicare's unfunded liabilities approach $48 trillion, making the shortfall almost twice as large as Social Security's. Worse, that estimate likely understates the true size of Medicare's problems. The Patient Protection and Affordable Care Act (ACA) made a number of changes to the program designed to reduce its cost, resulting in a projected net reduction in Medicare spending of $416.5 billion over 10 years, and more in the years beyond that.[5] Those savings projections are incorporated in the latest trustees report. Call that the optimistic or best-case scenario.

81

Many observers, including the CBO and Medicare's own actuaries, are skeptical that those anticipated savings will really happen. If they do not, Medicare could be in even worse shape.

The Medicare Program

Officially designated Title XVIII of the Social Security Act, Medicare was enacted in 1965 along with Medicaid, as the capstone of Lyndon Johnson's Great Society. At the time, it was viewed as a compromise measure, falling short of the universal health care system sought by many liberals. Today, it is often touted as the model for a government-run single-payer system.

Beyond the politics, more than 52 million seniors are currently part of the Medicare program, making it by far the largest U.S. government-run health care program. Indeed, Medicare payments account for fully 20 percent of all U.S. health care spending, giving the program enormous power with the U.S. health care market.[6] Decisions made about how Medicare pays doctors and hospitals or the services it covers reverberate throughout the entire health care system.

Although most people think of Medicare as a single program, it actually has several parts, with different benefits, funding sources, and enrollment requirements.

Medicare Part A: Medicare Part A covers care in a hospital, nursing home, or hospice, with benefits declining on the basis of length of stay. Nearly all Americans are automatically enrolled in Medicare Part A, whether they like it or not, on their 65th birthday. In fact, participation in Medicare Part A is a requirement for receipt of Social Security benefits. That is, individuals who decline to enroll in Medicare Part A can be denied any future Social Security benefits and can even be forced to repay any Social Security payments that they have already received. In addition, some nonelderly individuals with disabilities or chronic kidney disease have the option of enrolling in Medicare Part A. In 2013, approximately 52 million people were covered under Medicare Part A.[7]

Medicare Part A is financed through a 2.9 percent payroll tax (3.8 percent for individuals with incomes over $200,000 per year or with family incomes over $250,000. For those higher-income earners, the tax also applies to nonwage income, such as rents, dividends, interest, and capital gains).

There is a $1,260 deductible under Medicare Part A for each spell of illness. In addition, there is a $315 copayment per day after a hospital stay of more than 60 days. That copayment increases to $630 per day after 90 days. After 150 days, Medicare provides no further benefit.

Medicare Part B: Medicare Part B covers physician and outpatient care and associated services, such as durable medical equipment (for example, the motorized scooters that are ubiquitously advertised on TV); prosthetics and orthotics; laboratory services; preventive services, including vaccines (such as flu shots); and ambulance services.

Enrollment in Part B is voluntary. However, individuals who do not enroll on their 65th birthday may be required to pay a late enrollment penalty. That penalty is equal to 10 percent of the monthly premium for each year that a person could have otherwise been enrolled. That penalty must be paid every year after enrollment. For example, a person who waits until age 70 to enroll would be subject to a penalty of 50 percent, or $52.45 per month given today's premiums.[8] Thus, every year, that person would have to pay an additional $629.40 over and above his or her premiums.

In addition, individuals under the age of 65 who are receiving disability-based Social Security benefits are eligible for Medicare Part B after a two-year waiting period, as are most individuals suffering from chronic kidney disease. Medicare Part B is voluntary. Individuals age 65 or older may choose to enroll in the program by paying the monthly premium. Individuals under age 65 who are eligible for Medicare Part A because of disability or chronic kidney disease may also choose to enroll in Medicare Part B.

As indicated above, Medicare Part B is partially paid for through premiums. However, premium payments don't come close to providing sufficient funding. Therefore, the majority of funding for Medicare Part B comes from general government revenues. This year, Medicare Part B will cost taxpayers $205 billion.[9]

In 2013, approximately 52 million Americans were covered under Medicare Part A.[10] Slightly fewer Americans, 48 million, were enrolled in Medicare Part B. Of those, roughly 33 million received Part B reimbursed services last year.[11]

Medicare Part C: Medicare Part C is better known as the Medicare Advantage program. Under the program, Medicare contracts with private insurance companies to provide benefits under Medicare Parts A, B, and D (discussed next), as well as some additional benefits, such as vision care, dental, and extra days in the hospital. The benefits may vary considerably depending on the plan, but they must include all standard benefits provided under traditional Medicare. Those plans may offer traditional fee-for-service coverage, but they are more likely to be either managed care (HMOs) plans or preferred provider organizations. The plans may vary copayments and deductibles. They may also charge additional premiums. The choice of plan is up to the individual participant. However, some areas of the country may have very limited options.

Medicare Part D: The most recent addition to Medicare is Part D, which covers prescription drugs. Coverage is provided through private insurers, authorized by Medicare. As with Medicare Part B, enrollment is voluntary. However, individuals who do not enroll on their 65th birthday may be required to pay a late enrollment penalty, unless they have coverage under a Medicare Part C plan that offers prescription drugs.

Although the reimbursement structure under Part D is standardized (discussed next), participants have a wide choice of plans that vary greatly in their formularies (that is, the drugs they offer) and cost-sharing requirements (how much recipients must pay out of pocket). Participants pay a premium for coverage. However, as with Part B again, the premiums are far short of the money needed to fully finance the benefits, meaning that additional funding is needed from general revenues. This year, that general revenue portion will top $59 billion.[12]

The basic reimbursement structure for Medicare Part D is a complex plan often described as a "donut hole," although the hole will ultimately be phased out under the Patient Protection and Affordable Care Act. As originally designed, a Medicare recipient enrolled in the standard version of the prescription drug plan would pay a deductible of $250. Thereafter, Medicare would pay 75 percent of the costs between $250 and $2,250 in drug spending. The patient would pay the remaining 25 percent of those costs. The patient then encounters the notorious donut hole. For drug costs over $2,250 but under $3,600 in out-of-pocket spending, the patient must pay 100 percent of the costs. After that, the prescription drug plan kicks in again and pays 95 percent of costs over $3,600.[13]

However, the ACA ever so slowly closes that donut hole. Starting in 2011, a slow reduction in the amount that seniors have to pay out of pocket within the donut hole began, eventually reducing that amount from the current 100 percent to 25 percent by 2020. Part of the cost of filling the donut hole will be borne by pharmaceutical companies, which are required to provide a 50 percent discount on the price of brand-name drugs. That provision's cost to drug companies has been estimated at approximately $42.6 billion over 10 years.[14] The remaining 25 percent reduction in out-of-pocket costs will come from federal subsidies. For generic drugs, the entire out-of-pocket cost reduction is through subsidies.

An Ocean of Red Ink

As noted earlier, Medicare is facing future shortfalls of almost $48 trillion and possibly even higher. It should be obvious that unless the Medicare system undergoes serious systematic reform, disaster looms. Unfortunately, the reforms currently being discussed in Washington are unlikely to address the system's fundamental flaws.

Medicare's financial woes can be traced to three factors: demographics, technology, and third-party payment.[15]

First, as we saw when discussing Social Security, America is growing older. The baby boom generation is aging, and life expectancy is increasing. In 1965, when Medicare was established, the average American lived just over 70 years. Today, life expectancy has risen to over 78 years. By 2025, Americans can expect to live approximately 80 years, on average, even without any major new life-prolonging medical breakthroughs.[16]

Moreover, in 1965, a person who reached age 65 could expect to live an additional 14.6 years. That figure has now risen to 18.7 years, and it will continue to rise. As a result, by 2040, the proportion of Americans over the age of 65 will increase from 14 percent of the population to almost 21 percent. The number of Americans over the age of 70 will almost double.[17] Americans age 85 and older are now the fastest-growing segment of the population.[18] With medical breakthroughs and new technology, we can expect life expectancy to continue to increase, leading to even greater numbers of elderly citizens.

As a result, the CBO estimates that over the next 10 years, the number of Medicare enrollees will increase by one-third—approaching 72 million Americans.[19]

The older people become, the more, and more expensive, health care they consume.[20] Individuals over the age of 65 see physicians nearly twice as frequently as do younger Americans, and they enter the hospital twice as often.[21] Average per capita health care spending is approximately three times higher for the elderly than for the nonelderly, and the rate of increase in such spending for the elderly is nearly three times that for the nonelderly.[22] In general, half of a person's lifetime health care expenses are incurred after age 65.[23] As the number of elderly people continues to grow, Medicare expenses will continue to increase.

Second, medical treatments and technologies exist today that were not even dreamed of when Medicare was conceived. Those new treatments and technologies have saved lives and increased the quality of life, but they have also undeniably increased the cost of health care.[24]

Social Security's future costs are simply a matter of the number of seniors plus a formula for benefits. Medicare's costs, on the other hand, are also determined by the overall cost of health care. And that cost has been rising faster than overall inflation for years (Figure 6.1).

Figure 6.1

RISING HEALTH CARE CONSUMPTION PER CAPITA,
1960–2013

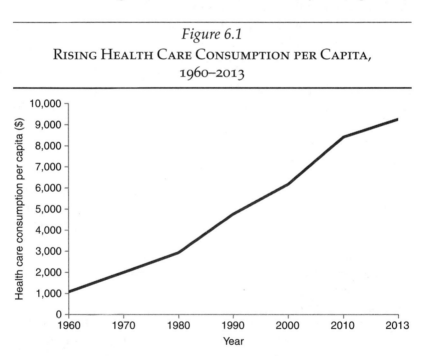

SOURCE: Centers for Medicare & Medicaid Services, "National Health Expenditure Data for 1960–2013."

As a result, per-enrollee costs in the program have been rising faster than per capita gross domestic product (GDP), at an average of 1.7 percentage points since 1985 (see Figure 6.2).[25] With the cost of benefits per recipient rising and the number of recipients also rising, that is a clear case of losing money on every transaction and trying to make it up through volume.

Figure 6.2

COST PER ENROLLEE AND TOTAL ENROLLMENT,
1987–2013

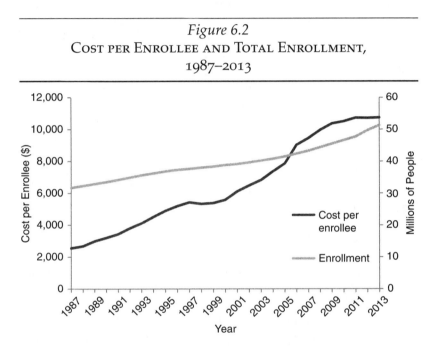

SOURCE: Centers for Medicare & Medicaid Services, "National Health Expenditure Data for 1960–2013."

There is some hope that the rise in health care spending may be slowing. Since 2010, health care expenditures have risen at an average of just 3.9 percent, compared with an average of 8.4 percent since 1970.[26] As a result, Medicare spending per beneficiary has grown by just 1 percent annually since 2010, slower, in fact, than either inflation generally or in GDP growth.[27]

But health care economists are unable to say why that slowdown has occurred or how long it will continue. Until recently, many thought the primary factor was the recession, which traditionally holds down health care spending. However, recent evidence suggests that the slowing of health care costs began before the recession and has continued even after it ended. That may mean that there are other, unidentified factors behind the slowdown (contrary to some liberal commentators, no evidence exists to suggest that Obamacare has had more than the most marginal effect), so there is some slender hope that costs can stay under control for some time to come. On the other hand, Medicare's trustees believe that the slowdown is a temporary phenomenon and project that Medicare outlays will average 6.39 percent growth over the next decade.[28]

Finally, while Medicare (and Medicaid, as discussed in Chapter 7) is at the mercy of overall health care costs, those problems are exacerbated by a fee-for-service system under which neither providers nor consumers have incentives to control costs. Medicare suffers from the problems inherent in any third-party payment system. Numerous studies have demonstrated that individuals will consume more, and more, expensive health care services if someone other than the consumer is bearing the cost. That is why Medicare utilization is roughly 50 percent higher than for private health insurance, even if you adjust for factors like age and medical conditions.

The deductible levels for Medicare are extremely low. Under Medicare Part B, for example, the deductible is a low $147, although there is a 20 percent copayment. The deductible under Part A is somewhat higher, $1,260 on the first 60 days of each hospital stay. A copayment is also required for hospitalization for more than 60 days. Over 90 percent of seniors have some form of supplemental insurance, including employer-sponsored retiree-covered insurance, Medicare Advantage, Medicaid, and Medigap that cover all or part of the deductibles and copayment.[29] For instance, studies have shown that seniors with Medigap use about 25 percent more services than Medicare enrollees who have no supplemental coverage.[30]

Although the deductibles for Part B have been indexed since 2005, they remain far below what they would be if they had been indexed to inflation since inception, and they remain too low to act as an effective restraint on overuse of health care services (Figure 6.3).

Figure 6.3
ACTUAL MEDICARE PART B DEDUCTIBLE VS. DEDUCTIBLE
INDEXED TO INFLATION, 1966–2014

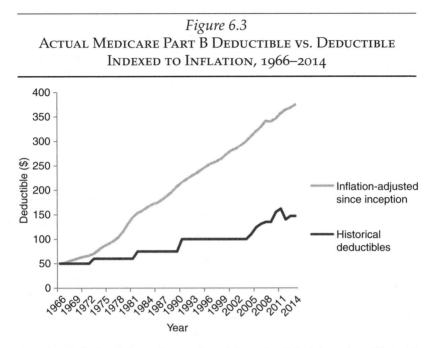

SOURCE: Calculated from data in Social Security Administration, "Annual Statistical Supplement to the Social Security Bulletin, 2011," SSA Publication no. 13-11700, February 2012; Bureau of Labor Statistics, "Monthly Labor Review and Labor Statistics," U.S. Department of Labor.

Thus, recipients pay very little out of their own pockets for Medicare services and have little incentive to be good consumers and avoid unnecessary expenses or seek the best deal for their dollar.

As a result of those factors, Medicare is careening toward bankruptcy. In fact, as Table 6.1 shows, three of the four parts of Medicare are already running deficits.

Let's start with Medicare Part A. In 2013, Part A spent roughly $31 billion more on benefits than it took in through the taxes intended to finance it. The problem of a growing elderly population is exacerbated because Medicare Part A suffers from the same inherent problems as do other pay-as-you-go systems, including Social Security. In theory, Medicare Part A is supposed to be funded through the Hospital Insurance portion of the payroll tax, currently

2.9 percent for employer and employee combined. In a pay-as-you-go system, today's benefits to the old are paid by today's taxes from the young. Tomorrow's benefits to today's young are to be paid by tomorrow's taxes from tomorrow's young. A pay-as-you-go structure is an intergenerational transfer from younger workers to older retirees.

TABLE 6.1
MEDICARE PROGRAM DEFICITS, 2013 (IN BILLIONS)

	Tax Income	Expenditures	Shortfall
Part A	$ 235.1	$ 266.2	$ 31.1
Part B	$ 63.1	$ 247.1	$ 184.0
Part D	$ 9.9	$ 69.7	$ 59.8
Total	$ 308.1	$ 583.0	$ 274.9

SOURCE: *2014 Annual Report of the Boards of Trustees of the Federal Hospital Insurance and Federal Supplementary Medical Insurance Trust Funds* (Baltimore: Centers for Medicare & Medicaid Services, July 28, 2014), Table II.B.1.

Like a chain letter or a pyramid scheme, the Hospital Insurance Trust Fund depends on a large pool of workers paying into the system for each recipient taking out of the system. Unfortunately, the ratio of workers to recipients has been steadily declining. Today, there are 3.2 covered workers for each Medicare beneficiary. By 2030, when today's workers have retired and our children are in their prime working years, there will be only 2.3 covered workers for each beneficiary (Figure 6.4).[31]

If the benefits paid to each recipient approximated the amount that that worker had previously paid in taxes, there would be no problem. However, Medicare Part A recipients currently receive significantly more in lifetime benefits than they pay in contributions (Figure 6.5).[32]

As noted, Medicare Part A is currently paying out more in benefits than it is collecting in payroll taxes, and it is relying on previously accumulated surpluses in the Medicare Trust Fund to cover the shortfall. By 2030, those surpluses will be exhausted, and Medicare Part A will no longer be able to meet its commitments.[33] That outcome actually represents a slight improvement in trust fund solvency, resulting from changes implemented under the Patient Protection and Affordable Care Act and the slowdown in health care cost growth, which as described previously is mostly due to the effects of the recession (Figure 6.6).[34]

Figure 6.4
WORKER-TO-BENEFICIARY RATIO, 2000–2085

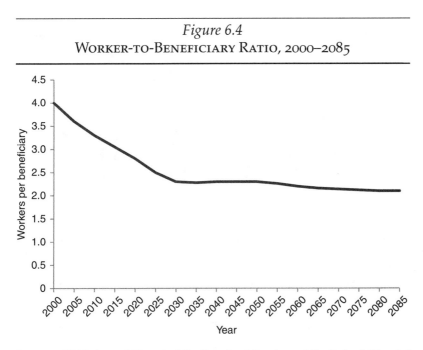

SOURCE: *2014 Annual Report of the Boards of Trustees of the Federal Hospital Insurance and Federal Supplementary Medical Insurance Trust Funds* (Baltimore: Centers for Medicare & Medicaid Services, July 28, 2014), Figure III.B4.

However, most observers remain skeptical about how much of those savings will actually materialize. More important, as with Social Security, Medicare's trust fund is simply an accounting measure, not an actual asset that can be used to pay benefits. What really counts is the program's cash flow, which, as noted, is negative. And, as shown in Figure 6.7, that cash flow will stay negative forever.[35] Overall, Medicare Part A's unfunded future liabilities approach $2 trillion.

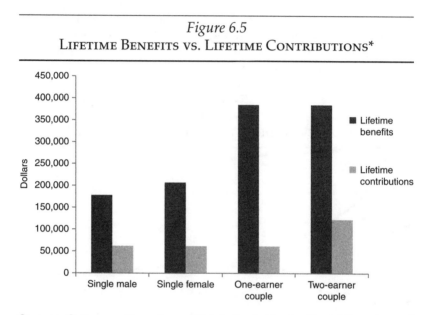

Figure 6.5
LIFETIME BENEFITS VS. LIFETIME CONTRIBUTIONS*

SOURCE: C. Eugene Steuerle and Caleb Quakenbush, "Social Security and Medicare Taxes and Benefits over a Lifetime: 2013 Update," Urban Institute, November 2013.

NOTE: *For beneficiaries earning the average wage and retiring at age 65.

The problems with Medicare Part B are no less serious. Approximately 73 percent of Medicare Part B is funded from general federal revenues, while about 25 percent is financed through premiums paid by beneficiaries. Since the program began, premiums have increased by a staggering 3,500 percent.[36] Still, those premiums have not been close to enough to pay for the program's benefits. Last year, they fell far short. Even including the taxation of benefits, a $185 billion shortfall occurred, requiring general revenues to contribute the difference.

Driven by the structural flaws noted earlier, from 2001 to 2011, total spending under Medicare Part B has grown at an average annual rate of 11.1 percent, and spending per enrollee has grown at a rate of 9.2 percent.[37] However, some recent signs of hope have appeared, as the overall slowing in health care costs has translated into slower Medicare growth. As a result, Part B spending grew at just 4.4 percent on average from 2010 to 2013, while per enrollee spending increased at an average rate of less than one percent.[38] Whether or not that slowdown will continue is a matter of much debate.

Figure 6.6
Projected Year of Part A Trust Fund Insolvency, 2002–2014

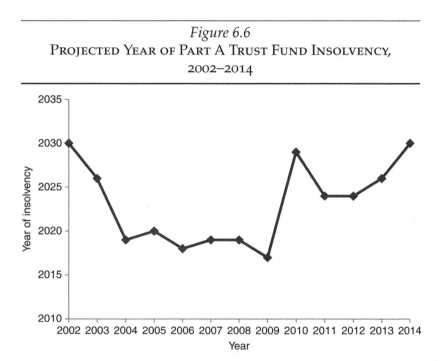

Source: Patricia A. Davis, "Medicare: Insolvency Projections," Congressional Research Service, July 3, 2013, Table 1; *2014 Annual Report of the Boards of Trustees of the Federal Hospital Insurance and Federal Supplementary Medical Insurance Trust Funds* (Baltimore: Centers for Medicare & Medicaid Services, July 28, 2014), Table II.E1.

Medicare Part C does not run a cash-flow deficit because of its structure, as payments are made out of the Hospital Insurance (HI) and Supplementary Medical Insurance (SMI) Trust Funds; those payments did cost $145.8 billion in 2013.[39] Roughly 24 percent of payments made from the HI Trust Fund are for Part C, and that component accounts for roughly 20 percent of payments from the SMI Trust Fund.[40]

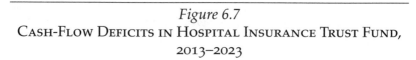

Figure 6.7
CASH-FLOW DEFICITS IN HOSPITAL INSURANCE TRUST FUND, 2013–2023

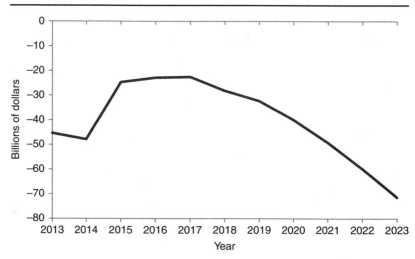

SOURCE: *2014 Annual Report of the Boards of Trustees of the Federal Hospital Insurance and Federal Supplementary Medical Insurance Trust Funds* (Baltimore: Centers for Medicare & Medicaid Services, July 28, 2014), Table II.E1.

And, although Medicare Part D has actually cost somewhat less than originally projected—shocking for a federal program—it nevertheless faces unfunded liabilities of more than $14 trillion. Although the ACA calls for savings elsewhere in the Medicare program, it actually increases spending under the prescription drug program by $42.6 billion, mostly by closing the donut hole.

Adding everything up, the total unfunded liabilities under all parts of the Medicare program, run to more than $47.6 trillion (Table 6.2). And that's the good news.

Table 6.2
MEDICARE INFINITE HORIZON UNFUNDED
LIABILITIES (TRILLIONS)

Part A	$1.90
Part B	$31.50
Part D	$14.20
Total	$47.60

SOURCE: 2014 *Annual Report of the Boards of Trustees of the Federal Hospital Insurance and Federal Supplementary Medical Insurance Trust Funds* (Baltimore: Centers for Medicare & Medicaid Services, July 28, 2014), Table II.E1.

As noted, the ACA made a number of changes to the program designed to reduce its cost.[41] The health care bill anticipates a net reduction in Medicare spending of $416.5 billion over 10 years.[42] The health care law would also bring in additional payroll tax revenue through a 0.9 percent increase in the Medicare payroll tax for single individuals with incomes over $200,000 or $250,000 for a couple, and the imposition of the tax to capital gains and interest and dividend income if an individual's total gross income exceeds $200,000 or a couple's income exceeds $250,000.[43]

But there is ample reason to doubt that the projected Medicare savings will occur. The CBO itself cautions that "it is unclear whether such a reduction in the growth rate of spending could be achieved, and if so, whether it would be accomplished through greater efficiencies in the delivery of health care or through reductions in access to care or the quality of care."[44]

For example, a new "productivity adjustment" would be applied to reimbursements to hospitals, ambulatory service centers, skilled-nursing facilities, hospice centers, clinical laboratories, and other providers, resulting in an estimated savings of $196 billion over 10 years.[45] There would also be $3 billion in cutbacks in reimbursement for services that the government believes are overused, such as diagnostic screening and imaging services. And beginning next year, the "utilization assumption" used to determine Medicare reimbursement rates for high-cost imaging equipment will be increased from 50 percent to 75 percent, effectively reducing reimbursement for many services.[46] That change is expected to reduce total imaging expenditures by as much as $2.3 billion over 10 years.[47] Other Medicare cuts include freezing reimbursement rates for home health care and inpatient rehabilitative services and $1 billion in cuts to physician-owned hospitals.[48]

The actuaries at the Centers for Medicare & Medicaid Services (CMS) claim that "neither of these update reductions is sustainable in the long range, and Congress is very likely to legislatively override or otherwise modify the reductions in the future."[49]

CMS offers an alternative projection based on more realistic payment assumptions in the long range, and finds that the unfunded liability of the overall Medicare program is closer to the levels reported in 2009 than to those in the 2010 report.[50] Using those alternative measures suggests that Medicare's unfunded liabilities could run as high as $89 trillion.

The reality is probably somewhere between the trustees optimistic scenario and CMS's worst-case one. Any way you look at it, Medicare is drowning in a sea of red ink.

Inefficiency and Inadequacy

Despite Medicare's financial crisis, making a case for the program's current structure might be possible if all that spending was buying quality health care, but the evidence overwhelmingly suggests that it is not.

Perhaps the clearest indication of that was found by the Dartmouth Atlas Survey, which uses Medicare data to provide comprehensive information and analysis about national, regional, and local markets, as well as individual hospitals and their affiliated physicians. The project uses those data to examine the relationship between health care use and outcomes in Medicare, asking questions such as, Do patients in high-spending areas start out sicker than patients in low-spending areas? Do they have better health outcomes? Do they report being more satisfied with their health care?

With over 20 years of intensive research, the project found that a higher volume of care does not actually produce better outcomes for patients. Patients in high-spending regions do not receive more "effective care," nor do they receive more "preference-sensitive care" (elective surgical procedures that have both benefits and risks, where patient preferences should determine the final choice of treatment). It also found that death rates in areas with less capacity and less use are not higher than death rates in areas where there is much higher capacity and use.[51] Most importantly, for the Medicare program, the project estimated that 30 percent of current health care spending is wasted.[52] The findings suggest that there is ample room to make Medicare more efficient without adversely affecting the health or happiness of beneficiaries, and that the program as it is currently constructed is wildly inefficient.

A separate study estimated that for 16 of 40 indicators, Medicare enrollees receive recommended care less than two-thirds of the time.[53] Other studies have found that Medicare does not provide better health care for the elderly than would private insurance. For that matter, there is not even a great deal of evidence that Medicare is better than no insurance at all. A 2009 study published in the *Journal of Health Services Research* found "the change in the trajectory of overall health status for the previously uninsured that can be attributed to Medicare is small and not statistically significant. Medicare coverage at age 65 for the previously uninsured is not linked to improvements in overall health status."[54] Similarly, a study by Amy Finkelstein and Robin McKnight for the National Bureau of Economic Research concluded that "Medicare did not play a role in the substantial declines in elderly mortality that immediately followed the introduction of Medicare."[55]

Perhaps the reason is, as the Medicare Payment Advisory Committee found: "Historically, Medicare payment systems have created little or no incentive for providers to spend additional resources on improving quality. Medicare's payment systems are not generally based on quality; payment is usually the same regardless of the quality of care. In fact, undesirable outcomes (e.g., unnecessary complications) may result in additional payments, and sectors with more-than-adequate payments may have little incentive to improve quality."[56]

Options for Reform

Fortunately, nearly everyone agrees that Medicare's current path is unsustainable. As President Obama put it, "Those of us who care deeply about programs like Medicare must embrace the need for modest reforms—otherwise, our retirement programs will crowd out the investments we need for our children, and jeopardize the promise of a secure retirement for future generations."[57]

However, that is where agreement ends. How to reform Medicare remains the subject of intense and divisive debate. Among the most frequently discussed options are to reduce reimbursement rates, to create the Independent Payment Advisory Board (IPAB), to increase payroll taxes, to raise premiums, and to raise the eligibility age.

Reduce Reimbursement Rates

Traditionally, the answer to rising Medicare costs has been to attempt to squeeze providers by enacting price controls, reducing reimbursement rates, or both. Virtually the entire history of the Medicare program has been a litany of one form or another of price controls, and recent developments continue down that well-worn path. The ACA cuts $415 billion through reductions in reimbursement rates in the next decade, accounting for almost 60 percent of the total estimated Medicare cuts.[58] Although it is admittedly unlikely to ever become law, the president's 2015 budget continues to rely on cuts to provider payments for the vast majority of Medicare savings; his budget envisions more than $354 billion in further cuts to provider payments, dwarfing the savings from proposed structural reforms to Medicare.[59]

Such cost controls have managed to reduce provider reimbursements to the point where many providers now receive 80 percent of the fee that private insurance pays and, under current law, would eventually plummet to 26 percent of private health insurance levels by 2086.[60]

Those provider cuts have had two major results. First, some of the program's costs have been shifted to the private insurance market. Studies suggest that between 12 percent and 23 percent of Medicare underpayment is shifted to private payers, although less cost shifting occurs in regions with highly competitive markets.[61]

Second, evidence is growing that Medicare price controls put at risk access to services and the quality of care. Enrollment in Medicare and access to care are not the same thing, and recently an increasing number of doctors are refusing to take new Medicare patients. A 2010 survey from the American Academy of Family Physicians found that 13 percent of its members did not accept Medicare patients at all in 2009, whereas only 5 percent did not accept new patients with private insurance.[62] A survey from the American Medical Association found that nearly one-third of physicians surveyed currently restrict the number of Medicare patients in their practice; the top two reasons they gave were that Medicare payment rates are too low, and that the ongoing threat of future payment cuts makes Medicare an unreliable payer.[63]

That trend may be accelerating. According to CMS, 9,539 physicians who had previously accepted Medicare opted out of the program in 2012. That's about two and a half times the number dropping out of the program in 2009.[64]

Squeezing waste and inefficiency out of the system would be a good thing, and some providers have certainly made a fortune by gaming the system.[65] But most proposals to cut provider payments are not really about *that*. Rather, such proposals are a covert attempt to reduce the benefits provided under Medicare, while shifting the blame for that reduction from politicians to the providers themselves. Rather than deny Medicare coverage for a procedure, the reimbursement cuts simply make it uneconomical for doctors and hospitals to provide it. The result is the same, but the blame is deflected.

That is not to say that some Medicare services and benefits shouldn't be eliminated, but provider cuts are an inefficient, blunt instrument for accomplishing that end.

Empower IPAB

The ACA goes even further down the path of reducing provider payments through the creation of the IPAB.[66] That new government entity, a 15-member panel appointed by the president, is not—as some conservatives have alleged—a death panel. It has no authority to determine whether a particular Medicare patient will receive a particular procedure. The panel will not be voting on whether grandma receives a hip replacement. However, that does not mean that IPAB's decisions may not limit the availability of that hip replacement.

According to the ACA, beginning in 2018, the annual growth in Medicare spending per capita is supposed to be no higher than the growth in GDP plus 1 percent. That is, if GDP grows at 3 percent, per capita Medicare spending could grow no more than 4 percent. Although at that rate this would fall far short of what is necessary to solve the program's future shortfalls, it is significantly lower than the program's traditional growth rate. In years when per capita Medicare spending exceeds that target growth rate, IPAB is required to submit a legislative proposal to Congress for how to bring spending back below the limit. Thus, if GDP grew at 3 percent while Medicare grew at 6 percent, IPAB would have to find ways to reduce per capita Medicare spending by two percentage points.

Similar to the way in which the Base Realignment and Closure Commission operated in the 1980s and 1990s, Congress could block IPAB's recommendations if both the House and Senate affirmatively voted to do so in their entirety. Congress could not amend the recommendations or pick and choose from among them. If either the House or Senate voted to uphold the recommendations, or if either chamber did not vote on them within 75 days, the recommendations would automatically go into effect.

Given Congress's demonstrated inability to make Medicare cuts that approach is not entirely unreasonable.[67] Still, major constitutional questions remain about whether Congress can delegate its responsibilities in that way.

Equally important, IPAB is likely to have a significant effect on the availability of care. IPAB is prohibited from making any recommendation that would "ration care," increase revenues, or change benefits, eligibility, or Medicare beneficiary cost sharing (including Medicare premiums).[68] That leaves IPAB with few options beyond reductions in provider payments, even beyond those already anticipated.

In fact, as Figure 6.8 shows, if per capita Medicare spending is truly limited to 1 percent above GDP growth, and if that reduction is accomplished entirely through reimbursement cuts, Medicare will pay physicians less than Medicaid by 2020, and, by midcentury, will be reimbursing providers barely half as much as private health insurance, well below the actual cost of providing care.[69]

Figure 6.8

CMS's Illustrative Comparison of Relative Medicare, Medicaid, and Private Health Insurance Prices under Current Law, 2000–2085

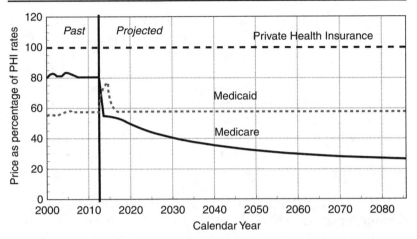

Source: Figure from Centers for Medicare & Medicaid Services, "Projected Medicare Expenditures under Illustrative Scenarios with Alternative Payment Updates to Medicare Providers," May 18, 2012.

In effect, physicians will be losing money every time they treat a Medicare patient. As previously noted, falling reimbursements are already driving providers out of the Medicare system. No wonder then that Richard Foster, the government's chief actuary, testified before Congress that the cuts likely resulting from IPAB could cause "serious" problems for patient access to care.[70]

Hospitals and other institutional health care providers will also be hit hard. CMS actuaries estimate that if the cuts projected in Figure 6.8 occur, 15 percent of hospitals and nursing homes could operate at a loss by 2019, and that number could surge all the way to 40 percent by the middle of the century.[71] Although some of those money-losing providers could merge with other operations or could be bought out, some will simply close. Hospitals in rural areas or inner cities, which are especially dependent on Medicare payments, are most at risk.

101

The result would soon be Canadian-style waiting lists in the United States. There would be health care rationing by effect, even if not actually by law.

Increase Payroll Taxes

It is theoretically possible to keep the Hospital Insurance Trust Fund solvent by radically increasing the payroll tax. But the increase would have to be quite large, taking an enormous toll on the American economy and employment. According to the Medicare trustees' *2014 Annual Report*, the current Medicare payroll tax would have to be increased from 2.9 percent (3.8 percent for incomes above $200,000) to at least 3.7 percent in order to restore Medicare Part A to solvency through 2088.[72] That would be a 28 percent increase, bringing the entire payroll tax to 16.1 percent (and that doesn't even consider any payroll tax hike that may result from Social Security's problems.)

It is also important to note that any future payroll taxes would come on top of the increases already enacted in the Patient Protection and Affordable Care Act. The law increased the employee's portion of the Medicare payroll tax by 0.9 percent for families making more than $250,000 a year (and for individuals making more than $200,000).[73] That increase would make the total Medicare rate 3.8 percent on every dollar of income over those thresholds. Most troubling, the revenues generated from that payroll tax increase are not even being used to fund Medicare but are instead funneled over to finance the ACA.

Past payroll tax increases are indicative of the effect a payroll tax increase would have on the American economy. A study by economists Aldona and Gary Robbins estimated that the payroll tax increases from 1985 to 1990 cost at least 900,000 jobs and reduced the U.S. gross national product by $25 billion per year.[74] More recently, the CBO estimated that allowing the temporary payroll tax reduction to lapse, which effectively increased rates from their temporarily lower levels by two percentage points, will reduce full "time" equivalent employment by 800,000.[75] Another study estimated that this expiration is likely to reduce real GDP growth by 0.6 percent.[76] Among country members of the Organization for Economic Cooperation and Development, the total tax rate was found to be the most important variable in determining the long-term unemployment rate.[77] Moreover, it is important to note that those payroll tax increases were smaller than the ones that will likely be needed to keep the Hospital Insurance Trust Fund solvent.

And all of that would still deal with only the shortfall in one portion of Medicare. Even if payroll tax hikes completely wiped out the unfunded liabilities of Medicare Part A, Medicare Parts B and D would still be running significant deficits. In fact, Medicare overall would still face a future shortfall of roughly $46 trillion.

Payroll tax increases should be discarded as a potential solution to reforming Medicare because an increase would cause significant economic damage while also failing to address any of the inherent problems with the Medicare program.

Raise Premiums

Any effective Medicare reform is likely to require at least some seniors to pay more for the benefits they receive. One way to do that is by increasing the premiums that they pay, notably for Medicare Parts B and D, which are partially financed through those premiums.

Medicare Part B premiums were means-tested starting in 2007, and the ACA introduced means testing for Part D. As a result, seniors earning more than $85,000 in 2014 will pay slightly higher premiums for Medicare Parts B and D, continuing with small increases in premiums up the income ladder, with the highest threshold being $214,000 for an individual.

Those premium hikes affected fewer than 5 percent of seniors. However, a more general premium hike would be necessary to deal with the program's financial shortfalls (Figure 6.9). For example, premiums will already have to increase 49 percent by 2023 just to keep pace with Medicare spending. To increase premium revenue to the point where it covers 35 percent of Part B costs, premiums would have to drastically increase by 108 percent.[78]

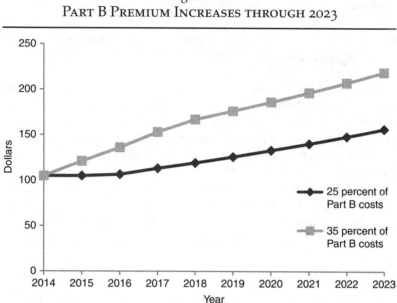

Figure 6.9
PART B PREMIUM INCREASES THROUGH 2023

SOURCE: *2014 Annual Report of the Boards of Trustees of the Federal Hospital Insurance and Federal Supplementary Medical Insurance Trust Funds* (Baltimore: Centers for Medicare & Medicaid Services, July 28, 2014), Tables V.E2, V.E3.

NOTE: Additional premium increases in the 35 percent scenario are phased in until 2018; thereafter premiums are at a level that would finance 35 percent of program costs.

Premium hikes, or at least means-tested increases, are likely to be part of any Medicare reform, especially in the short run. However, it is important to recognize that premium increases are not a substitute for structural reform. Indeed, in the absence of structural reform, premium increases simply throw more money into the current failing system.

True, premium hikes are fairer than tax increases, because the person consuming the services is the one paying for them. But if we are simply going to chase every higher cost with more money, we will eventually reach a limit on what seniors can pay. Already, the average senior pays $1,536 per year.[79] For moderate- and low-income seniors, that represents a substantial burden.

Raise the Eligibility Age

Successful Medicare reform will also likely include significant future benefit cuts—not reductions in provider payments, but actual reductions in the benefits that seniors receive. One of the most frequently discussed ways to reduce benefits is to gradually increase the age at which an individual becomes eligible for Medicare. When Medicare began, its eligibility age was 65, the same as for Social Security. However, the retirement age for Social Security is currently scheduled to be gradually increased to age 67 by 2022. Under current law, the eligibility age for Medicare will remain at 65.

Medicare's eligibility age should be gradually increased in a way similar to Social Security and then indexed to increases in longevity. The CBO estimated that gradually raising the eligibility age by two months each year starting in 2014 would save Medicare $162.5 billion through 2021.[80] The increases would mirror those in Social Security; after 2020, the eligibility age in both programs would be the same, reaching 67 in 2027 and indexed to increases in longevity after that (Figure 6.10).

That change would represent a step in the right direction, but it would still solve only a tiny fraction of Medicare's problems. More is needed.

Structural Reforms

The necessary reform of Medicare must address the program's fundamental structural flaws. The program cannot continue as a third-party, first-dollar payer for the health care needs of a growing elderly population. Spending additional revenues will simply throw good money after bad. Reducing reimbursement rates will not yield significant savings, but it has and will compromise the quality of care. There is, quite simply, no way to preserve Medicare as we know it.

Figure 6.10
Eligibility Age, Social Security and Medicare, 1998–2025

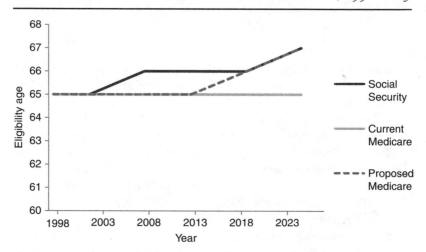

Source: Congressional Budget Office, "Options for Reducing the Deficit: 2014 to 2023," November 2013.

For example, there is no reason why Medicare should be separated into distinct parts, each with separate funding mechanisms, cost-sharing requirements, and other rules. That structure of having separate components is mainly historical, reflecting the structure of private insurance as it existed in the 1960s, which had separate silos for hospital care and physician care. (In fact, the first insurance plans covered only hospitalization.) Since then, the norms in private insurance have changed, and a single deductible for all medical services is typical.

Merging Medicare Parts A, B, and D into a single unified structure represents a logical starting point for any structural reforms to follow. That approach already has broad cross-ideological support. For example, scholars from the liberal Urban Institute and the Commonwealth Fund have endorsed the concept.[81] The Obama administration has shown interest in the idea, as have some Republican reformers.[82] A similar proposal was made by the Bowles-Simpson Commission.[83]

Creating a single unified structure would certainly simplify Medicare for beneficiaries and make it easier for seniors to understand.

The new structure would do better at internalizing some of the costs of medical care use for more beneficiaries; low-use seniors who are generally healthy would see a slight increase in out-of-pocket spending. That higher level of cost sharing, combined with greater transparency (due to the simpler, unified structure) would lower some aspects of health care use that do not add a significant amount of value. On the other side of the coin, merging those components would also do more to protect the most medically needy seniors from exorbitantly high health costs, reducing their risk of medical bankruptcy.

Merging the separate components would also mitigate the need to purchase supplemental insurance like Medigap, which places additional financial burdens on seniors and increases the inequality in the level of care seniors enjoy.

That step would go some way to making the program more efficient by reducing excess health care use and lowering total cost, while also protecting the most vulnerable and sickest beneficiaries.

Having restructured Medicare into a single unified program, there are two other possible approaches to further reform instituting premium support and vouchers and reforming the cost-sharing structure.

Institute Premium Support or Vouchers

One approach to Medicare reform would shift the program from its current defined-benefit structure to a defined-contribution system. As the program is currently constructed, Medicare beneficiaries are guaranteed access to a set of health care services that will be covered and paid for by the government. In that type of system, the government has very little control over costs; as health care costs and the number of beneficiaries grow, so too does the cost of Medicare. Defined-contribution plans, on the other hand, specify the level of government support that will be given to beneficiaries, who then use it to obtain health insurance or to pay for health care directly.

Defined-contribution approaches to Medicare reform generally fall into two categories: premium support or vouchers. Both would shift more control and decisionmaking to seniors, establishing a link between contributions and benefits but with some major differences, particularly in how they determine the level of support the government provides to beneficiaries. In premium-support proposals, like the one found in the most recent iteration of Paul Ryan's "Path to

Prosperity," the level of government support is based on the cost of a benchmark private insurance plan that covers a defined basket of services. In that system, the level of support would not depend on which plan beneficiaries chose to enroll in: if they chose to enroll in a plan that cost less than the premium support amount, they could keep the cost savings; whereas if they selected a plan that cost more than the premium support amount, they would have to make up the difference in the form of premium payments.

That mechanism would incentivize beneficiaries to choose cheaper, more cost-effective plans, because they have a significant degree of cost exposure, whereas insurers would be encouraged to provide lower-cost plans to attract more enrollees. In that system, both providers and beneficiaries would seek to constrain costs, unlike today where both parties have little incentive to use services efficiently or judiciously. In more recent premium-support proposals, the amount of support would grow with the benchmark plan, as opposed to being indexed to inflation.

In a voucher system, the government contribution is not defined by the cost of coverage, and there is no set of health services that plans must offer to be eligible for the voucher; beneficiaries can use the voucher to purchase a health insurance plan of their choice, purchase health care directly, or deposit the money into a dedicated health savings account. That level of support would then be indexed to some economic measure, whether inflation or economic growth, rather than the cost of a benchmark plan.

Vouchers and premium support also differ in where the federal support payments go: with vouchers they go directly to Medicare beneficiaries who then decide how they can best be used, whereas with premium support systems, seniors must choose from a list of approved private insurance plans, and the government payment goes directly to those insurance companies.

Premium-support systems usually impose many more restrictions than vouchers. Premium-support proposals generally require all plans to provide a minimum basket of services, equivalent to either current Medicare or another benchmark plan, in order to be eligible to enroll Medicare beneficiaries and receive government premium-support payments. Plans in that system would be constrained in their ability to compete effectively, because they would be obligated to offer the same benefits package, which limits the amount of

108

flexibility and innovation at their disposal as they attempt to attract enrollees. Because they cannot vary the services covered in their plans in any significant way, insurance providers are much more limited in ways to innovate and to compete for enrollees.

Vouchers impose no such restrictions, and beneficiaries would not be required to purchase health insurance; they could instead deposit the money into a dedicated health savings account. The fear of losing so many potential customers would pressure insurers to make their plans more affordable and would prevent them from engaging in a race to the bottom, where few medical services are covered.

House Ways and Means Committee chairman and former vice presidential candidate Rep. Paul Ryan of Wisconsin is perhaps the politician most commonly identified with both vouchers and premium support. He first introduced a proposal for changing Medicare to a defined-contribution structure in his 2008 "Road Map for America's Future."[84] In every iteration of his budget proposal since then, Ryan has shifted further and further away from vouchers and toward premium support.

In his original plan from 2008, for example, Ryan proposed that when Americans currently age 55 or younger become eligible for Medicare, they receive a payment approximately equivalent to per capita Medicare spending that would then be indexed to the average of overall inflation and medical inflation. Those voucher payments would also be adjusted for risk and geographic area. Low-income beneficiaries would receive contributions to medical savings accounts that could be used to pay for coinsurance and deductibles, limiting their out-of-pocket cost exposure.

His proposals in subsequent years moved further and further away from that concept, with Ryan adopting many of the more restrictive features of premium-support plans. In fact, Ryan took pains to refer to his 2012 proposal as premium support and not vouchers, pointing to the fact that the government payments would go directly to private health insurers instead of beneficiaries.[85] The 2012 proposal would have established a Medicare exchange, much like those created in the Affordable Care Act, in which private insurance plans would have to comply with a standard for benefits, in this case set by the Office of Personnel Management. Plans in the exchanges would have to issue insurance to all beneficiaries who applied and would have to charge the same premiums for all enrollees of the same age.

The most significant evolution in his recent plans was the change in determining the amount of government support, and how that payment was indexed to grow over time. Like its more recent predecessors, the 2014 Ryan proposal would establish a Medicare exchange, but in this version, the level of premium support would be determined by the second-least-expensive private insurance plan in a region, or traditional fee-for-service Medicare, whichever was lower.[86] For the first time, traditional fee-for-service Medicare would remain as an option for enrollees, which introduces a raft of problems. Allowing traditional Medicare to continue would undermine much of the competition that is supposed to rein in costs in the system; if traditional Medicare was not consistently one of the most affordable options, supporters of the traditional program would lobby to increase taxpayer subsidies to make it more attractive or "affordable," allowing Medicare to undercut private insurance options despite offering an inferior product and severely weakening competition.

It is also worth noting that none of Ryan's proposals would take effect until a decade after they were proposed, meaning current enrollees would be stuck in ineffective fee-for-service Medicare and be denied the benefits of greater choice and higher-quality health care. Meanwhile, the fiscal position of Medicare would continue to deteriorate, adding to the burden for current and future workers with higher deficits and higher taxes.

A far better approach would give every retiree the right to opt out of the Medicare system by receiving a voucher equal to the average annual per capita expenditure under Medicare. That voucher could be used to purchase private insurance or to make contributions to a medical savings account. Such a reform would give seniors more control over their medical care, while also encouraging them to be more cost conscious. The amount of the voucher could be risk adjusted to reflect beneficiaries' age, sex, geographic location, and health status. Older and sicker individuals would receive a larger voucher than younger and healthier beneficiaries and would not find themselves in a situation where they were unable to afford care.

Enrollees who wish to purchase a plan more expensive than the adjusted voucher amount would pay the difference in the form of an additional premium, and enrollees who choose a lower-cost plan could deposit unspent voucher funds into a health savings account that could be used for out-of-pocket medical expenses and future premiums. Unlike today's Medicare program, vouchers would give enrollees an incentive to choose efficient health plans that proide access to quality care. The vouchers would also allow them to escape the increased rationing and reduced quality of care under Medicare and choose the private coverage and services they prefer.

Allowing seniors to opt out of Medicare with vouchers would enable Congress to effectively constrain the growth in Medicare spending. Each year, Congress would be able to adjust total Medicare outlays for the growth in enrollees and overall inflation. That change would put Medicare outlays on a reasonable and sustainable path.

Congress should provide vouchers to current Medicare enrollees, not just future enrollees. Delaying implementation would deny enrollees the benefits of greater choice and higher-quality health care, while at the same time Medicare's fiscal health would continue to deteriorate, contributing ever-increasing amounts to the annual budget deficit.

Reform the Cost-Sharing Structure

A second approach would leave the basic defined-benefit structure of Medicare unchanged but would gradually convert the program to more of a catastrophic insurance program.

Once Medicare was unified into a single program, it would have a single deductible that should initially be set high enough to deter overuse. The CBO estimates that even an annual deductible of $550, with a coinsurance rate of 20 percent for amounts above that deductible for all services, would save $10 billion in 2015 and $110 billion through 2020.[87]

That initial deductible should gradually be increased to at least $2,500 and possibly as high as $10,000. At the same time, the outer limits of coverage should be increased to provide a clear stop loss against catastrophic costs. In many ways, that change would be the inverse of the current Medicare program, which has very low deductibles but fails to cover long-term care.

Because the increase in deductibles would be phased in gradually, younger workers would have time to save against the higher out-of-pocket expenses that they would incur. To make such saving easier, they should have the opportunity to contribute to a personal account similar to those suggested for Social Security (see Chapter 5).

In 1999, Harvard University's Martin Feldstein calculated that personal savings accounts financed by worker deposits averaging 1.4 percent of wages would be enough to make up Medicare's future funding shortfall.[88] Although it would almost certainly require a much higher contribution today, the basic idea remains sound.

A simulation developed for the National Center for Policy Analysis by Andrew Rettenmaier and Thomas Saving of Texas A&M looked at a scenario under which Medicare Parts A, B, and D are combined into a single insurance plan.[89] Every Medicare recipient then has a base deductible, or defined cost-sharing requirement, indexed to grow at the same rate as overall per capita Medicare spending. The initial base deductible used in the projections for the study is $2,500, which is in the neighborhood of a senior's current combined average spending for an individually purchased Medigap policy and for out-of-pocket Medicare expenses. Current beneficiaries would pay current deductibles and premiums, but the $2,500 indexed figure would serve as a maximum cap. For future beneficiaries, each individual's total Medicare cost sharing will equal the base deductible plus the amount of the annuity that individuals purchase for themselves.

In addition, workers are required to contribute 4 percent of their income to a health insurance retirement account. When they enroll in Medicare at age 65, beneficiaries will use their account balances to purchase an annuity paying an annual fixed sum.

They found that by midcentury, spending for the reformed Medicare program would be 20 percent to 35 percent less than the current program.[90] In fact, even if contributions to the health insurance retirement accounts were included, total spending for Medicare would be less than the spending for the current program. At the same time, average-income workers entering the labor market today will have annuities that pay an amount equal to 29 percent to 59 percent of their projected spending on Medicare-covered services at the midpoint of their retirement years.[91]

Although the study is dated, it does show that a personal savings plan could replace at least a significant portion of the current Medicare program. At the very least, this approach deserves further study.

Conclusion

The Medicare system is no longer sustainable in its current incarnation as a first-dollar insurance plan. Demographics, technology, and the incentives of a third-party payment system will continue to drive up costs.

The most commonly suggested solutions—raising the payroll tax, increasing premiums, and reducing reimbursements—will not address the program's inherent, structural flaws. Instead, Congress should increase the age of eligibility, raise deductible levels, and allow the elderly to opt out of the system. Various options for making that transition include vouchers, premium support, and the use of personal savings accounts. All of those mechanisms would begin the transformation of Medicare to a backup catastrophic insurance program.

Only through such a revolutionary transformation of the Medicare system can we ensure that the elderly will continue to have access to the highest-quality health care, without bankrupting their children and grandchildren.

7. Medicaid: Strike Two for Government Health Care

Given the enormous problems facing Medicare, it is easy to ignore those of its little brother, Medicaid, the government's second-largest health care program. Yet Medicaid's finances are nearly as bad, adding to the federal deficit today, with huge shortfalls looming on the horizon. And, unlike Medicare, Medicaid is also an increasing burden for state budgets.

That burden is almost certain to grow for both the federal and state governments as Medicaid expands as part of the Patient Protection and Affordable Care Act (ACA). Medicaid is already one of the largest government programs, with an average monthly enrollment of 58 million people and total spending of $432 billion. The Congressional Budget Office (CBO) estimates that, under the ACA, as many as 16 million additional Americans will enroll over the next decade.[1]

At the same time, the current Medicaid program is rife with problems, not the least of which is that it fails in its mission of providing quality health care to the poor.

The Medicaid Program

Medicaid was created in Title XIX of the Social Security Act in 1965; it is a means-tested entitlement program financed jointly by federal and state governments designed to assist states in providing medical assistance to eligible needy persons. In its current form, the federal government provides financing and a set of national guidelines, while the states administer the program. Within the established federal guidelines, states set eligibility standards, determine what services will be covered, and set payment rates for providers. There is a significant degree of variation among the states in all three channels; no two state Medicaid programs are exactly alike. A person who is eligible for Medicaid in Florida might not be eligible in Texas, and services covered by Medicaid in Oregon might not be covered in Washington.

Medicaid in every state is required to cover a number of mandatory services, including long-term care, laboratory and x-ray services, inpatient hospital care, and others. States also have the option to cover additional services like physical therapy and hospice services. The program also imposes restrictions on the extent to which states can require beneficiaries to share in the cost of those services; there are limits to the amount of cost sharing states can impose, what groups can be required to pay, and what must be covered without any form of cost sharing.

Originally, there were two aspects to Medicaid eligibility, *categorical restrictions* and *financial requirements*; both determinants have been significantly relaxed, or done away with altogether, in recent years. In the early years of the program, categorical restrictions ensured that Medicaid served a target population of the truly vulnerable: the elderly, the disabled, children from very low-income families, and their parents. Eligibility was based in large part on receipt of cash assistance under other federal programs like Aid to Families with Dependent Children. In recent years, eligibility has shifted away from those categorical restrictions and has become increasingly determined by income thresholds, and this trend will continue even further under the ACA.

The federal government and the states share the responsibility for funding Medicaid. States pay providers or managed-care organizations for Medicaid costs and then report those payments to the Centers for Medicare & Medicaid Services. The federal government pays for a percentage of the costs of medical services by reimbursing each state, known as the Federal Medical Assistance Percentage (FMAP), and it varies by state, according to a calculation that is in part based on per capita income. FMAPs were temporarily boosted in the stimulus package but have since returned to their normal levels. In 2013, the FMAP ranged from a low of 50 percent in 14 states to a high of 73.43 in Mississippi.[2] Although the FMAP for the newly eligible population will be changed under the ACA, those already eligible will continue to operate under the current rates.

When analyzing the Medicaid program, it is important to remember that its beneficiaries are not uniform; there are actually four different groups that can be eligible for Medicaid: children, adults, the elderly, and disabled individuals. Those groups have very different health care needs, and the per capita spending per enrollee varies accordingly; federal benefit payments ranged from $1,530 per child beneficiary to $11,350 per elderly beneficiary.[3] As Figure 7.1 shows, although adults and children make up the majority of enrollees (74 percent), they account for a far smaller share of expenditures (35 percent).[4] Disabled and elderly beneficiaries account for the vast majority of program expenditures, even though they make up a much smaller proportion of enrollees, because they are much more likely to have chronic conditions and higher overall use of health care services. There is even more variation when one considers that the composition of enrollees also varies significantly from state to state; although elderly and disabled enrollees constituted only 16 percent of total enrollees in Arizona in 2010, in Kentucky and Pennsylvania, they were 35 percent.[5] The Medicaid programs in those two states have very different needs; a rigid, uniform reform imposed by the federal government is unlikely to substantially address the diverse problems those state Medicaid programs face. Comprehensive Medicaid reforms should account for the diversity of Medicaid enrollees and their health care needs.

Figure 7.1
Medicaid Enrollment and Expenditure by Eligibility Group

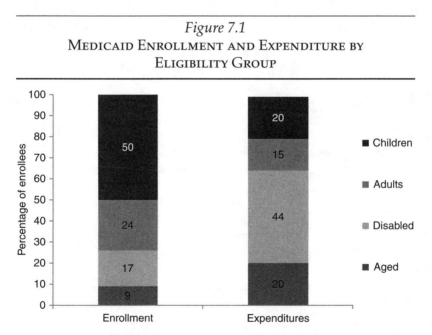

Source: Department of Health and Human Services, "2012 Actuarial Report on the Financial Outlook for Medicaid."

Medicaid has expanded significantly since its establishment, from a targeted program that served a small, vulnerable population to one of the largest government programs. In 1970, five years after its creation and after enough time had elapsed for all of the provisions to take effect, 14 million Americans were enrolled in the program, and total spending was only $5.1 billion.[6] Today, average monthly enrollment is roughly 58 million people, and total spending is more than $430 billion (Figure 7.2).[7] The program has shifted away from the targeted, categorical restrictions on eligibility to define eligibility more in terms of income, which has led to an expansion in enrollment and a surge in program costs in recent years.

Figure 7.2
ENROLLMENT AND COST GROWTH, 1970–2011

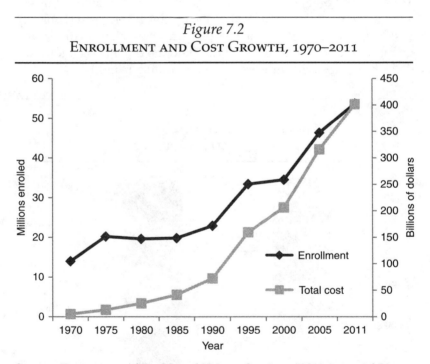

SOURCE: Department of Health and Human Services, "2012 Actuarial Report on the Financial Outlook for Medicaid."

The CBO projects that Medicaid spending will increase at an annual rate of 7 percent over the next 10 years. Federal Medicaid costs are estimated to more than double from $265 billion to $545 billion by 2023—by which point average monthly enrollment will have swelled to 72 million (Figure 7.3).[8]

Figure 7.3
PROJECTED COST AND ENROLLMENT GROWTH, 2013–2024

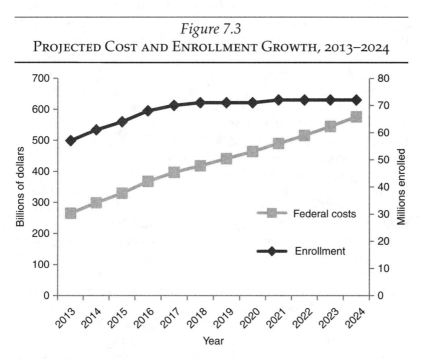

SOURCE: Congressional Budget Office, "Updated April Budget Projections—Medicaid Baseline Projections," April 14, 2014.

Although the ACA will contribute significantly to the looming surge in Medicaid costs and enrollment, Medicaid costs were already projected to surge before the law was enacted; the 2008 actuarial report of the Department of Health and Human Services projected that total Medicaid costs would more than double from 2007 to 2017.[9] Even before the ACA, Medicaid was set to place an unsustainable burden on federal and state budgets, and the inherent flaws in the program prevented it from providing access to quality care for beneficiaries. The ACA does nothing to address any of those problems; instead, it merely serves to expand a deeply flawed program.

Impact on State Budgets

Even before the program was expanded under the ACA, Medicaid represented the single-largest portion of total state spending, accounting for 25.8 percent of total state spending in FY 2014.[10] To put that in perspective, education, the second-largest state budget item, accounted for just 19.5 percent of state spending.

Rising Medicaid spending poses a particular problem for state budgeting because, unlike the federal government, almost all states are required to balance their operating budgets. That means that states facing an increasing burden of Medicaid spending will have to raise taxes, or else Medicaid will eventually squeeze out funding for other priorities like schools and roads.

Unfortunately for states, the mechanisms they would usually use to find savings in their Medicaid programs (cutting provider payments, reducing benefits, or restricting eligibility) will be either ineffective or prohibited in the coming decade. Provider payments in many states are already so low that many doctors no longer take Medicaid patients, so further cuts would put beneficiaries' access to care at risk.

States also have incentives to shift people onto the Medicaid rolls, and they are deterred from moving beneficiaries off the rolls because of the way the program is financed. States can leverage additional federal funding through the expansion of their Medicaid programs; each dollar they spend on their Medicaid programs receives matching federal funds. To illustrate, a state with a 50 percent match (the lowest rate) could expand its program by $2 million, and the federal government would pay $1 million. That leverage works in reverse when a state tries to cut Medicaid costs: they must cut at least $2 from the Medicaid program (depending on the FMAP) to achieve $1 in state budget savings. Because of the unique financing structure of Medicaid, states have virtually no incentive to make their programs more efficient and cut costs in their Medicaid programs unless they are absolutely forced to by budgetary concerns.

The federal funding mechanism creates even more problems under the ACA (see below) since the enhanced match for expansion population makes a state facing budget constraints more likely to seek savings from the traditional Medicaid population, which is more vulnerable. Essentially, because a state is only covering 5 percent of the costs of expansion in 2017, it would have to cut $20 of expenditure to save the state $1. As the matching rate declines to 90 percent, this figure falls to $10. In the traditional population, with lower matching rates, it would have to cut $2.32 on average (using 2015 matching rates) to save $1. Thus the expansion could actually put some of the more vulnerable groups (children, disabled) in traditional Medicaid at more risk of future program cuts.

Medicaid Expansion under the ACA

Under the ACA, Medicaid is scheduled to expand even further in the next decade, further straining state budgets, causing federal spending to skyrocket, and relegating even more Americans to low-quality health care.

Starting this year, individuals with income levels below 138 percent of the federal poverty level would be eligible, mainly affecting the childless adult population. The federal government would pick up much of the cost for that expansion population, at least initially, financing all of the costs for the first three years, before gradually phasing down to 90 percent. Initially, that Medicaid expansion was essentially mandatory—all federal Medicaid funding would be withdrawn if states refused to expand—but in *National Federation of Independent Business v. Sebelius*, the Supreme Court ruled that the Medicaid expansion "violates the Constitution by threatening States with the loss of their existing Medicaid funding if they decline to comply with the expansion" and struck down the provision allowing the Department of Health and Human Services to withdraw existing Medicaid funds for failure to comply with the expansion.[11]

As a result, the Medicaid expansion is now optional, and a degree of uncertainty still exists as to how many states will refuse to expand their Medicaid program. So far, 27 states and the District of Columbia have expanded their programs in accordance with the ACA, although some have done so in conjunction with waivers that also introduced other reforms (Figure 7.4).[12] Some of the states

121

with the largest uninsured populations, such as Florida and Texas, have so far declined to expand, fueling uncertainty as to how many people will enroll because of the Medicaid expansion, and how much it will cost.

As of October 2014, roughly 9.68 million more Americans are enrolled in Medicaid than the average before expansion, but many of those were simply the result of normal churning within the Medicaid system, as well as the so-called "woodwork effect."[13] The "woodwork effect" is when people who were previously eligible but not enrolled in Medicaid join the program, perhaps because of outreach efforts related to the expansion. This "woodwork" population is not eligible for the enhanced federal match, only the traditional Medicaid matching rate.

Figure 7.4
STATUS OF MEDICAID EXPANSION IN THE STATES

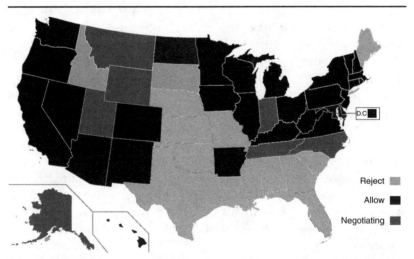

SOURCE: Kaiser Family Foundation, "Current Status of State Medicaid Expansion Decisions," December 17, 2014.

The CBO has revised its projections accordingly, regularly ratcheting downward its estimates of how many people will be added to the Medicaid rolls from a projected 17 million by 2020 before the Supreme Court's ruling down to a projection of roughly 13 million (Figures 7.5 and 7.6).[14]

Figure 7.5

CHANGE IN ENROLLMENT DUE TO MEDICAID EXPANSION, 2014–2022

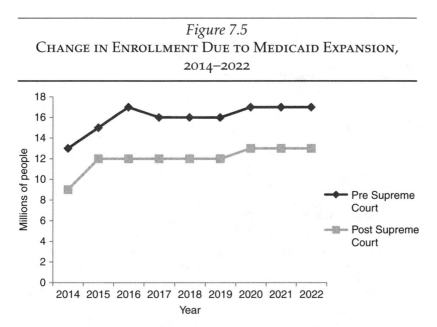

SOURCE: Congressional Budget Office, "Updated Estimates for the Insurance Coverage Provisions of the Affordable Care Act," March 13, 2012; Congressional Budget Office, "Effects on Health Insurance and the Federal Budget for the Insurance Coverage Provisions in the Affordable Care Act— April 2014 Baseline," April 14, 2014.

If Medicaid enrollment because of the ACA is not as high as originally forecast, that is bad news for those hoping that the ACA would lead to universal coverage. But it is actually good news for federal and state budgets. As it dropped its coverage projections, the CBO also reduced its estimate for ACA-related increases in Medicaid costs. The CBO now suggests that the ACA will increase Medicaid spending by $101 billion by 2024. That's still problematic, of course, but it is $316 billion less through 2022 than had been initially projected.[15]

Figure 7.6
CHANGE IN MEDICAID EXPANSION COSTS, 2014–2022

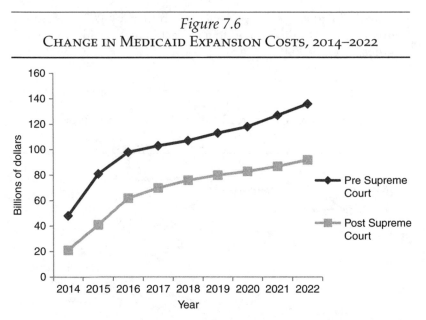

SOURCE: Congressional Budget Office, "Updated Estimates for the Insurance Coverage Provisions of the Affordable Care Act," March 13, 2012; Congressional Budget Office, "Effects on Health Insurance and the Federal Budget for the Insurance Coverage Provisions in the Affordable Care Act—April 2014 Baseline," April 14, 2014.

Fundamental Flaws of the Medicaid Program

Our enormous entitlement programs have two crucial recurring themes. First, they are driving the country toward bankruptcy. Second, in exchange for all we spend on them, they don't actually do a very good job. We saw that problem with Social Security, where the program, even if solvent, provides younger workers with a return far below what they could earn through private investment. We saw it with Medicare, where outcomes appear unrelated to the amount of money spent, and the program is developing increased access problems.

If anything, Medicaid may be an even more egregious example. Observers from across the political spectrum agree that, financing aside, Medicaid delivers poor quality care. Among the biggest problems are access to care, quality of care, and improper payments and fraud.

Access to Care

Contrary to what proponents of Medicaid expansion may wish, enrollment in the Medicaid program is not the same thing as having access to health care. Some characteristics of the program might limit beneficiaries actual access to a doctor; low reimbursement rates and bureaucratic headaches cause many doctors to limit the number of Medicaid patients they serve, or even refuse to take Medicaid patients at all. A recent analysis published in *Health Affairs* found that only 69.4 percent of physicians accept Medicaid patients compared with more than 80 percent of physicians who accept privately insured patients.[16] A study published in the *New England Journal of Medicine* found that individuals posing as mothers of children with serious medical conditions were denied an appointment 66 percent of the time if they said that their child was on Medicaid (or the related Children's Health Insurance Program [CHIP]), compared with 11 percent for private insurance—a ratio of 6 to 1.[17]

Even when doctors do still treat Medicaid patients, barriers to actual care remain, and Medicaid enrollees often have a harder time getting appointments and face longer wait times. One study found that among clinics that accepted both privately insured children and those enrolled in Medicaid, the average wait time for an appointment was 42 days for Medicaid and 20 days for the privately insured.[18] Enrollment in Medicaid is not synonymous with access to health care services because inherent flaws in the Medicaid program—from low reimbursement rates to more paperwork—erect barriers between enrollees and health care services. Even when they do get access to care, it is often of poor quality.

In an attempt to encourage more doctors to accept Medicaid, the ACA included a temporary two-year increase in the program's reimbursement rates. After costing taxpayers roughly $5.5 billion in 2013–14, that increase expired on January 1 of 2015. Some states are planning to tap their own taxpayers in order to extend the increased reimbursement, but others are unlikely to come up with the money to pay for the extension. In states that don't pony up their own money—covering an estimated 71 percent of Medicaid recipients—physician reimbursements could fall by as much as 47 percent.[19] That's not going to encourage doctors to sign up more Medicaid patients.

Yet, as noted above, the number of people on Medicaid will have increased significantly. It doesn't require an economic genius to realize what happens when increased demand meets reduced supply.

Quality of Care

Many studies have found that people enrolled in Medicaid receive lower-quality care and have worse health outcomes. A landmark study published in the *Annals of Surgery* examined outcomes for almost 900,000 individuals undergoing major surgical operations from 2003 to 2007. The University of Virginia study found that "surgical patients on Medicaid are 13 percent more likely to die than those with no insurance at all and 97 percent more likely to die than those with private insurance."[20] That trend of lower-quality care continues through numerous studies: Medicaid patients were found to have higher rates of surgical complications and were less likely to have cancer diagnosed at earlier, more treatable stages.[21] In almost every health outcome, Medicaid is outperformed by private health insurance.

By far the most important Medicaid study to come out in recent years is the Oregon Health Insurance Exchange study. The reason that study is so important is that it is the first randomized controlled study—often considered the gold standard of research—to examine the effects of insurance on health outcomes.

The opportunity for the study arose when Oregon determined that it had enough funds to provide health insurance to an additional 10,000 uninsured low-income adults—but 90,000 people wanted in. To be as fair as possible, the state held a lottery, and then it followed the participants over time to measure the effect of access to Medicaid. The study found that access to Medicaid increased health care use, and medical spending increased from $3,300 to $4,400 per person, but those increases were not reflected in health outcomes. As the authors concluded, "This randomized, controlled study showed that Medicaid coverage generated no significant improvements in measured physical health outcomes in the first 2 years."[22]

As lackluster as those results are, they are in all likelihood better than they would be in the country as a whole, since Oregon's reimbursement rates are higher than average, and more doctors accept new Medicaid patients. That extremely important study lays bare many of the inherent flaws of the Medicaid program, finding that health outcomes show no real improvement, while the poor incentive structure leads to excess use and increased costs. Those findings reinforce the need to fundamentally reform the Medicaid program to provide better-quality health care more efficiently and to call into question the benefits of expanding the current program as called for in the ACA.

Improper Payments and Fraud

As inefficient as spending taxpayer money on an inefficient program like Medicaid might be, a significant portion of that money does not even go to the flawed program but is instead the product of waste and fraud. According to the Centers for Medicare & Medicaid Services (CMS), the improper-payment error rate was 5.8 percent ($24.9 billion) in 2013, although the exact amount of supplemental payments is unknown because state reporting was incomplete.[23] The CMS estimate of 5.8 percent waste, while still significant, is probably optimistic; Malcolm Sparrow from Harvard has estimated that fraud and improper payments could be 20 percent of the cost of federal health programs, which would mean Medicaid waste of more than $85 billion a year.[24] Although it may not be impossible to know the precise level of fraud and waste in the program, we do know that it is pervasive; as the inspector general of the Department of Health and Human Services said, "Everywhere it looks the Office of Inspector General continues to find fraud."[25]

The high level of fraud is a result of the program's financing structure. The states administer the program and decide how much to spend, but the federal government pays most of the costs. That arrangement removes the incentive for state officials to deal with fraud and abuse; they bear few of the costs and capture little of the savings. To weed out the pervasive waste and abuse in Medicaid, the federal matching structure that finances the program needs to be reformed.

Reforming Medicaid

Ironically, even as Medicaid has been expanded under the ACA, there has been a growing awareness that the program is posing an unsustainable burden for both federal and state governments. Even President Obama has suggested that federal commitments to the states may have to be scaled back.[26] To date, most such proposals would simply move costs around, changing who pays them, but they would not fundamentally reduce long-term program costs.

Recently, however, some more fundamental and structural changes have been proposed.

Vouchers

One proposal that would fundamentally transform Medicaid would end the open-ended, entitlement structure of the program and convert it into a voucher program. Instead of the states paying providers, and the federal government reimbursing them for part of the costs, individuals would receive vouchers and would then be free to choose from a variety of health insurance and health care options. They would then be able to purchase traditional insurance or instead choose a high-deductible plan and deposit the balance of their voucher into a health savings account.[27]

Such a reform would shift the decisionmaking process away from federal and state governments, instead empowering beneficiaries. If individuals choose a more efficient, cheaper plan, they will have the option of saving the remaining amount of the voucher in a health savings account to defray potential health costs they may incur later. If they choose a plan that is more expensive, they will have to make up the difference between the voucher and the plan costs from their own funds. That increased responsibility and decisionmaking power will encourage individuals to choose cost-effective policies best suited to their needs, which would allow them to access better-quality care, while also reining in cost growth.

Vouchers would be set at a specified level initially, either comparable to per capita Medicaid spending or the cost of an equivalent private insurance plan, and then adjusted annually by some measure of inflation. One benefit of this reform proposal is that it would shift millions of low-income Americans from Medicaid to private insurance.

As described earlier, the Oregon study found no statistically significant physical health outcomes resulting from Medicaid coverage, and Medicaid patients have a much harder time getting appointments to see doctors than people with private insurance.[28] This reform would go some way to ending the two-tier health system that is currently in place, incorporating those low-income people into the higher-quality private health insurance market.

One potential concern with the proposal is that the government would still impose significant restrictions on the health care marketplace for this Medicaid population by requiring voucher plans to cover a certain basket of services, or to have a certain actuarial rating, much like the regulations seen with the health insurance exchanges in Obamacare. Such burdensome regulation could inhibit the competition and choice that are so essential to controlling costs. As we saw with the premium-support option for Medicare, plans in this system would be unable to compete effectively because they are obligated to offer what is essentially the same benefits package, which limits the amount of innovation they can pursue as they attempt to attract enrollees.

Another potential concern with a voucher program is that it would in some ways concentrate too much power at the federal level, as voucher amounts and essential benefits would likely be determined in Washington; states would have limited flexibility to innovate to determine best practices. It is also possible that it would create another inadvertent welfare trap: if the voucher amount is phased out with increases in earned income, poor people could face prohibitively high marginal tax rates, especially when the marginal tax rate effects of the program are combined with other means-tested welfare programs. That new welfare trap would then discourage this vulnerable population from working more hours or finding a better job, and it could ultimately have the perverse effect of actually locking the majority of this population into dependency for the foreseeable future.

Although the voucher reform would greatly improve the Medicaid program by increasing consumer choice, it also has its share of potential problems.

Block Grants

Block grants would be the most effective way to give states the maximum amount of flexibility, and they could reduce the growth of future Medicaid costs if properly structured. With the block grant, the federal government would give each state a lump sum each year for the entire program, allowing federal taxpayer costs to be directly controlled. Block-granting the program would have two budgetary effects.

First and foremost, that reform could generate significant budget savings for the federal government. The total amount of savings would depend on the initial level of funding, or benchmark year, and whether the amount would be indexed to inflation or another growth factor. Using a very conservative benchmark year of 2014 would establish a federal spending cap of $299 billion to be apportioned among the 50 states by Medicaid enrollment.

That is conservative because it includes the additional spending from higher Medicaid enrollment because of the recession and the first year of the Obamacare Medicaid expansion. A case could be made that the benchmark year should be set at pre-recession levels, in which case budget savings would be even greater. Using the 2014 levels as the baseline, block-granting Medicaid and keeping it at those levels through 2024 would save more than $1.5 trillion, with annual spending in 2024 being roughly $277 billion lower than it would be without the block grant.[29]

Some people argue that federal funding should be indexed to inflation, or some other factor like population growth or number of people below the poverty line, because otherwise the purchasing power of that Medicaid funding would dwindle over time, leading to a loss of services or diminished quality. Indexing the cap to inflation would allow federal funding to rise and fall in tandem with inflation, keeping the purchasing power of that federal funding more constant over time. That approach would significantly reduce budget savings, but it could also make it somewhat more palliative for states; the CBO projected that indexing the cap to inflation starting October 2015 would save $450 billion through 2023, so it would still achieve significant budget savings, albeit not nearly as much as a flat block grant would.[30]

Regardless of which year is chosen as the benchmark and what the amount is indexed to, if anything, significant savings would be achieved by the block grant simply through the elimination of federal administrative expenses, which are projected to be $226 billion over the next decade.[31]

Another benefit of converting to a block grant is that it would place Medicaid on a much more predictable, stable financial trajectory; in its current form, the growth in the program and the amount of federal funding available to states are unpredictable, adding to uncertainty for both states as they attempt to balance their budgets, and federal taxpayers concerned about the ever-increasing national debt.

The main nonbudgetary benefit of the block grant is that, if executed properly, it would imbue the states with the agency to design more cost-effective health care programs tailored to their different Medicaid populations. In Medicaid today, there is a perverse incentive for states to enroll as many people as possible in the program in order to capture as many federal dollars as possible; states have limited incentive to make their programs more effective or to pursue cost savings because they do not really see the benefits. Even if they had the motivation, states are too restricted in their ability to experiment with their Medicaid programs. They are at the mercy of the administration to obtain waivers from Medicaid rules governing what benefits they must cover, or restricting their ability to experiment with different cost-sharing schemes.

The current waiver system is overly burdensome. In some ways, the system inhibits states in their attempts to improve their Medicaid programs. Increased flexibility for the states is therefore an essential component of Medicaid reform. The effectiveness of the block grant approach can be seen in the success of the 1996 welfare reform, where the open-ended entitlement Aid to Families with Dependent Children was converted into a block grant. The reform reined in program costs that had been soaring in recent years while helping beneficiaries join the workforce and transition out of the program.

In his most recent House budget, Paul Ryan has proposed a block grant reform for the entire program, estimating that such a reform would save $810 billion relative to current policy over the next decade.[32]

With a fixed amount of federal funding and fewer federal regulations, states would have a strong incentive to make their programs more efficient and the ability to tailor their program to the specific needs of their Medicaid populations.

The block grant would enable the federal government to reduce federal Medicaid funding. Policymakers at all levels would benefit from having the program on a predictable path. States would be better able to plan how to best use their federal funding without having to worry about unforeseen cuts in federal matching rates. Medicaid's impact on federal deficits would be less subject to fluctuation, lending a degree of predictability to the medium-term fiscal outlook. At the same time, such reform would unleash the innovative power of the states, leading to a myriad of improvements in program administration and design that would make it more effective and cost efficient. The block grant reform is the best solution for Medicaid because of those two channels: significantly increased flexibility for states and substantial budget savings that would greatly improve Medicaid and make it fiscally sustainable.

Conclusion

If there is one thing we should have learned by now, it is that the government does a remarkably poor job of running a health care system. Medicaid is yet another example. Costs are rising, posing a significant problem for both federal and state governments.

At the same time, the evidence is overwhelming that Medicaid provides poor-quality health care to program participants. In fact, being enrolled in Medicaid may provide few benefits over being uninsured.

Expanding Medicaid under the ACA will only exacerbate the program's problems. Instead of expanding the program, we should be making fundamental changes to the program's structure in ways that will give states greater flexibility and that will allow for the experimentation that can reduce costs over the long term. As with so many other government programs, simply throwing more money at the problem will only make matters worse.

Medicaid, like Medicare and Social Security, is ripe for reform.

8. Obamacare: Little Bang, Lots of Bucks

One might have thought that, given the enormous debt and future obligations that this country is facing, we would avoid taking on yet another entitlement program. And not just *any* entitlement, but a massive new program whose future costs could rival those of Social Security, Medicare, and Medicaid. Like the hypothetical family that we started with in Chapter 1, Congress has decided to go on a spending spree despite being deep in debt.

In fact, our fiscal condition is worse now than when those other entitlement programs were enacted. As Figure 8.1 shows, in the first

Figure 8.1

AVERAGE ANNUAL BUDGET DEFICITS, FIVE YEARS AFTER PASSAGE

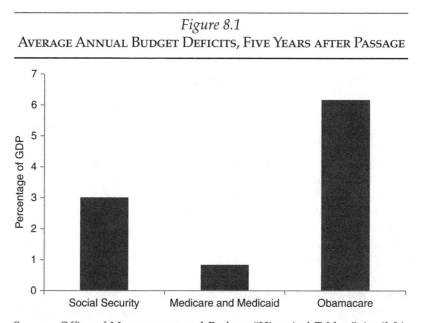

SOURCE: Office of Management and Budget, "Historical Tables," April 24, 2014, Table 2; Congressional Budget Office, "Updated Budget Projections: 2014 to 2024," April 14, 2014.

five years after Medicare and Medicaid became law in 1965, the average annual budget deficit amounted to less than 1 percent of the gross domestic product (GDP). Social Security was launched during the Great Depression, but in the five years that followed, average annual deficits were only 3 percent of GDP. But in the next five years following Obamacare's being signed into law, deficits are projected to total 5.5 percent.[1]

That is one reason that Charles Blahous, a former trustee of the Medicare and Social Security systems, describes the Patient Protection and Affordable Care Act as "the greatest act of fiscal irresponsibility ever committed by federal legislators."[2]

The Patient Protection and Affordable Care Act

The Patient Protection and Affordable Care Act (ACA), more colloquially known as Obamacare, was more than 2,500 pages and 500,000 words long.[3] In the years since its passage, various agencies of government have issued more than 70,000 pages of regulations and guidance to implement it.[4] It creates dozens of new agencies, boards, commissions, and other government entities.[5] Several parts of the law have been changed or postponed, often by executive order.[6] A few provisions have even been repealed or amended by Congress.[7] It has been both upheld and altered by the courts. Additionally, a great deal of misinformation, conjecture, and rumor has been circulating in both the mainstream and alternative media. No wonder, then, that many Americans remain confused by the law itself and its effect on them, their health plans, and their businesses. Despite the complexity of the law itself, and the well-reported difficulties of its implementation, the ACA boils down to five key components: (a) the individual mandate, (b) the employer mandate, (c) insurance regulations, (d) exchanges, and (e) subsidies and Medicaid expansion.

Individual Mandate: As of March 31, 2014, every American was required to have health insurance coverage that meets the government's definition of "minimum essential coverage." Those who don't receive such coverage through government programs, their employer, or some other group must purchase individual coverage on their own or pay a penalty. Last year, that penalty was 1 percent of the individual's adjusted gross income or $95, whichever is greater.[8] But it ramps up quickly, the greater of $325 or 2 percent of annual income this year, and the greater of $695 or 2.5 percent of annual income after that. In calculating the total penalty for an uninsured family, children count as half an adult, which means that in 2016 an uninsured family of four would face a minimum penalty of $2,085 ($695 + $695 + $347.50 + $347.50), prorated on the basis of the number of months that the person was uninsured over the course of the year.[9]

It is important to point out that simply having insurance is not necessarily enough to satisfy the mandate. To qualify, insurance would have to meet certain government-defined standards for "minimum essential coverage." That requirement is only logical. If a person could theoretically pay $1 for an insurance plan with a $10 million deductible, it would defeat the whole purpose of the mandate.

Many of the required benefits are common sense and are already included in nearly all insurance plans. They include outpatient care, emergency room treatment, hospitalization, and laboratory tests. Other benefits, however, are less common, and their inclusion is subject to greater debate. They include maternity and newborn care, mental health and substance abuse treatment, prescription drugs, rehabilitative and habilitative services, a wide variety of preventative and wellness services, chronic disease management, pediatric services, and dental and vision care for children. Beyond the specific benefits, plans are required to have an actuarial value (the average percentage of health care expenses that will be paid by the plan) of at least 60 percent. In addition, qualified plans must also comply with all the various insurance regulations included in the ACA.[10] Thus, the individual mandate is not just a mandate to have insurance but a mandate to have the specific type of insurance that the government has designed.

That provision, of course, was the subject of a major Supreme Court decision in 2012. In the case of *National Federation of Independent Business v. Sebelius*, the Court upheld the insurance requirement, not as a mandate, but rather as a tax on uninsured individuals.[11] Ironically, however, in upholding the mandate in that manner, Chief Justice John Roberts, who wrote the deciding opinion, was in effect saying that the mandate was a tax because it was so small that it would not actually force individuals to buy insurance. Roberts was effectively acknowledging that it is cheaper to "pay" than to "play." As we will see, that could lead to serious adverse-selection issues going forward.[12]

Employer mandate: The law also contains an employer mandate. Starting January 1, 2016, all businesses with 50 or more full-time employees must provide health insurance coverage to their workers or pay a penalty. The mandate was originally scheduled to take effect in 2014. However, in September 2013, President Obama, by executive order, postponed the implementation until 2015.[13] After another delay, employers with 50 to 99 workers now have until 2016, whereas those with 100 or more workers can avoid any mandate penalties by covering only 70 percent of workers in 2015.[14]

There are two possible ways for companies to calculate the penalty for failing to provide insurance—with companies required to pay the *lesser* of the two amounts. Under the first method, the company must pay a tax penalty of $2,000 for every person it employs full-time (minus 30 workers). Thus, a company employing 100 workers would be assessed a penalty of $140,000 ($2,000 × 70 workers). Alternatively, the company could pay $3,000 for each uninsured employee who qualifies for a subsidy through an exchange.

As with individuals, to satisfy the mandate, insurance must meet the government's definition of an acceptable plan. Employer-provided insurance (with a partial exception for self-funded plans under the Employee Retirement Income Security Act) must meet the same requirements as individual plans, fulfilling the "essential minimum benefits" package and all requisite insurance regulations.

Initially, this mandate is likely to affect relatively few companies. Roughly 96 percent of companies with more than 50 employees already provide health insurance.[15] And although many of the plans currently offered do comply with ACA requirements (for example, deductibles may be too high or they may not provide all the benefits specified), those plans are "grandfathered," meaning companies can keep them in place for now, but, as with individual plans, any "substantial change" invalidates the grandfathering. Therefore, many—if not most—employer plans will also have to change in order to comply with the mandate (discussed later).

Insurance regulations: The ACA imposes a host of new federal insurance regulations that significantly change the way the health insurance industry does business. Some of those regulatory changes have so far been among the law's most popular provisions, but many are likely to have unintended consequences.

136

Perhaps the most popular insurance reform allows parents to keep their dependent children on their policies until the children reach age 26.[16] A second popular reform prohibits insurers from imposing lifetime limits on benefit payouts.[17] In a similar vein, the law also bans "rescissions," or the practice of insurers dropping coverage for individuals who become sick.[18]

In addition, the law requires insurers to maintain a medical loss ratio (that is, the ratio of benefits paid to premiums collected) of at least 85 percent for large groups and 80 percent for small groups and individuals.[19] Insurance companies that pay out benefits in amounts less than the required proportion of the premium revenues must rebate the difference to policyholders annually beginning in 2011. That requirement is intended to force insurers to become more efficient by reducing the amount of premiums that can be used for administrative expenses (and insurer profits). Already, insurers have been forced to provide more than $1.59 billion in rebates to individuals and businesses.[20]

But perhaps the most significant regulatory reform is the ban on insurers denying coverage because of preexisting conditions. Under the Patient Protection and Affordable Care Act, insurers are prohibited from making any underwriting decisions based on health status, mental or physical medical conditions, claims experience, medical history, genetic information, disability, other evidence of insurability, or other factors to be determined later by the secretary of Health and Human Services (HHS).[21] Specifically, the law requires insurers to "accept every employer and individual . . . that applies for such coverage."[22]

Finally, there are limits on the ability of insurers to vary premiums on the basis of an individual's health. That is, insurers must charge the same premium for someone who is sick as for someone who is in perfect health.[23] Insurers may consider age in setting premiums, but those premiums cannot be more than three times higher for their oldest than for their youngest customers.[24] Smokers may also be charged up to 50 percent more than nonsmokers.[25] The only other factors that insurers may consider in setting premiums are geographic location and whether the policy is for an individual or a family.[26] These provisions started for children in 2010 and for everyone else on January 1, 2014.

It should be noted that although the ban on medical underwriting may make health insurance more available and affordable for those with preexisting conditions and may reduce premiums for older and sicker individuals, it will increase premiums for younger and healthier individuals (discussed later).

Overall, most of the law's insurance reforms have been among the more politically popular aspects of the new law. Although their ultimate effect may be small, helping fewer people than is commonly believed, they do address real problems. Any alternative to the ACA will also have to find ways to deal with these issues.

Exchanges: Health exchanges, rebranded as "marketplaces" by the Obama administration, were a technological "train wreck" throughout the fall of 2013, but they remain a key component of the ACA.

The exchanges are designed to function as clearinghouses, wholesalers, or intermediaries, matching customers with providers and products. Exchanges also allow individuals and workers in small companies to take advantage of the economies of scale, both in administration and risk pooling, currently enjoyed by large employers. Exchanges are also the mechanism through which individuals receive subsidies to help pay for insurance.

The legislation gave states the option of setting up an exchange, or, if they chose not to do so, the federal government would establish and operate an exchange in that state. States could also operate part of an exchange, leaving the federal government to operate the rest.[27] As it turns out, state decisions broke largely, but not entirely, along partisan lines. Thirteen states and the District of Columbia chose to operate their own exchanges, whereas the federal government ended up running—in whole or part—37 exchanges.[28] Some state-run exchanges have been a disaster, even among states that have been enthusiastic supporters of Obamacare since day one. Oregon's exchange has been such a failure that the federal government is stepping in to take over, and Maryland and Massachusetts may possibly follow suit.[29]

Subsidies and Medicaid expansion: With regard to the law's impact on the federal budget, the most important provisions are those designed to expand coverage by subsidizing it, either through government-run programs such as Medicaid and the Children's Health Insurance Program (CHIP) or through subsidizing the purchase of private health insurance. Of course, subsidies should be no surprise, since the number one reason that people give for not purchasing insurance is that they cannot afford it.[30] Still, the subsidies will be expensive.

As discussed in Chapter 7, states are able to increase eligibility for Medicaid as of last year, so that all individuals with income levels below 138 percent of the federal poverty level would be eligible for the program, an increase in eligibility that mainly affects the childless adult population.[31] The federal government will pick up much of the cost for that expansion population, at least initially, financing all of the costs for the first three years before gradually phasing down to 90 percent.[32]

To date, only 27 states and the District of Columbia have expanded their programs. Some of the states with the largest uninsured populations—Florida and Texas—have so far declined to expand, fueling uncertainty as to how many people will enroll because of the Medicaid expansion and how much it will cost.[33]

Individuals with incomes too high to qualify for Medicaid but below 400 percent of the poverty level ($88,000 per year) are eligible for subsidies to assist their purchase of private health insurance. According to the Centers for Medicare & Medicaid Services (CMS) and outside organizations such as the Kaiser Family Foundation, roughly 86 percent of the more than 8 million Americans who signed up for insurance through exchanges in the first round of open enrollment received a subsidy to help pay for their insurance.[34] This proportion increased throughout the open enrollment period; in early months, roughly 80 percent qualified for financial assistance. In the first month of 2015 open enrollment, this rate is even higher at 87 percent.[35]

A recent report from HHS found that federal subsidies paid for 76 percent of the premium amounts for people who qualified for them on the federal exchange.[36] That fact stokes fears that the cost projections could be underestimating how much the federal government is spending on exchange subsidies, which could affect future deficits. Worse, since it's possible that fewer than 2 million enrollees were previously uninsured, millions of Americans who were previously paying for their own insurance have now moved into a system, at least during the program's first year, where the government is paying most of the cost.

And it's not as though those subsidies are going only to the poor, who otherwise could not afford insurance. Although more generous to those earning 250 percent of the poverty line ($58,875 for a family of four), some amount of subsidy is available up to 400 percent of the poverty level ($94,200 for a family of four). In fact, taking into account various income disregards, some families with even higher incomes could receive a subsidy. The Congressional Budget Office (CBO) estimates that as many as 700,000 people with incomes of more than three times the poverty level will receive a subsidy next year.[37]

It is important to note that by the time this book is published the Supreme Court may have thrown out subsidies in those states that have a federally run exchange. As written, the ACA explicitly authorizes subsidies only through "an Exchange established by a State."[38] That means subsidies should not be available through federal exchanges. The language of the statute is clear, and the ever-loquacious Jonathan Gruber has stated that the law was set up that way to entice states into establishing their own exchanges.[39]

If the Court upholds the challenge in the case of *King v. Burwell*, some 5 million people in 36 states would lose their subsidies, meaning they would suddenly have to pay more, sometimes much more, for insurance. On the other hand, since it is an employee's receipt of subsidized coverage that triggers the employer mandate, businesses in those states would find themselves free of that burden. Moreover, individuals who, without subsidies, can no longer find affordable insurance would be exempt from the individual mandate. Elimination of the subsidies could also increase the likelihood of an "adverse selection death spiral." Lastly, a ruling against the subsidies would significantly reduce the program's overall cost. In short, if the Court rules that the ACA must be implemented as written, the entire program could unravel quickly.

The Court heard the case in March 2015 and was expected to rule by the end of June 2015, about the time this book is scheduled for release.

The Cost of Obamacare

In June of last year, the CBO announced that because of so many changes, postponements, and waivers to the law, it could no longer provide an accurate estimate of its cost or impact on the deficit.[40] Faced with an Obama administration that seems to unilaterally rewrite the law almost daily, the CBO essentially gave up trying to score it. Of course, maybe that is honest Washington budgeting for a change. We have a great big program that's going to spend a lot of money, but we really don't have any idea of how much.

Still, it is worth examining the history of the CBO's cost estimates for the ACA, their limitations and failures, and what those estimates portend for the program's ultimate cost and impact on the debt.

140

When the ACA was passed in 2010, the CBO scored the coverage provisions of the legislation, the Medicaid expansion and exchanges, as costing $938 billion over 10 years, from 2010 to2019.[41] That was, of course, highly misleading because almost all of the program's expenditures occurred after 2014. The CBO was therefore issuing a 10-year score that included just 6 years of spending. Now, four years later, the law is more or less fully implemented. The CBO's most recent ACA baseline puts the major coverage expansion programs' cost at $1.84 trillion from 2014 to 2024.[42] It is important to note that much of the increase in estimates since 2010 is simply due to the extended projection window.

In addition, attempts to compare year-over-year cost estimates run into problems given the law's frequent changes. In many cases, it is difficult to compare apples to apples. For example, when the Supreme Court made it optional for states to expand Medicaid (see Chapter 7), the CBO reworked its assumptions to take into account Medicaid participants in states that chose not to expand their programs. Estimated ACA costs have also risen and fallen in tandem with estimated insurance premiums.

For example, the most recent ACA baseline from the CBO, released in April, is roughly $165 billion lower over 10 years than the projection released two months earlier, a decline quickly touted by the program's advocates. However, the savings reduction almost exclusively results from the fact that initial insurance premiums were somewhat lower than the CBO predicted. Since subsidies are linked to premium prices, lower premiums reduce subsidy payouts. Therefore, if premiums remain low, the program's costs will indeed be lower than previously predicted. That is a big "if," however. For reasons that will be discussed, it is unlikely that premiums will remain below estimates in the future. If premiums rise significantly, so will the required subsidies, and therefore program costs.

Moreover, "lower" does not mean "low." Even taking the new CBO estimates at face value, the ACA will consume a far greater portion of GDP in 2015 than Social Security did five years after it became law.[43] In fact, you could add the cost of Medicaid five years after passage to the cost of Social Security five years out, and it would still be less than the cost of Obamacare after 5 years (measured as a percentage of GDP). Only Medicare is comparable (Figure 8.2).

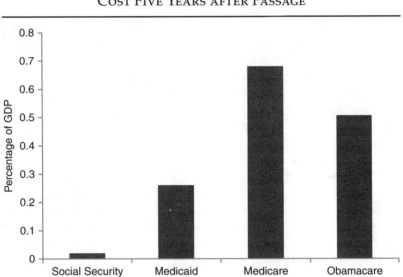

Figure 8.2
COST FIVE YEARS AFTER PASSAGE

SOURCE: Congressional Budget Office, "Updated Budget Projections: 2014 to 2024," April 14, 2014; Office of Management and Budget, "Historical Tables," April 24, 2014, Table 13.1.

If the ACA grows in the out years in the same—often unanticipated—ways as other entitlements have, the future costs could be even greater than for other programs.

It is also important to remember that such CBO estimates significantly understate the actual costs of the health care law. For instance, the initially projected cost failed to include discretionary costs associated with the program's implementation. The legislation does not provide specific expenditures for those items; it simply authorizes "such sums as may be necessary." Because the costs are subject to annual appropriation, and the actions of future Congresses are difficult to predict, putting a precise figure to the amount may be impossible.

However, the CBO suggests that they could add as much as $100 billion to the 10-year cost of the bill.[44] For example, HHS has passed out $4.4 billion in grants to states last year, and plans to spend an additional $1.2 billion by the end of this fiscal year. The law also includes between $5 billion and $10 billion over 10 years for the Internal

Revenue Service to enforce aspects of the law, and an additional amount for the Department of Health and Human Services. The operation of exchanges in the 37 states where they are being run by the federal government is expected to be $3.5 billion for 2013–2014 and more in subsequent years.[45] None of that money is included in ACA cost estimates.

In addition, estimates of the ACA's impact on the budget deficit double count both Social Security taxes and revenue and savings from Medicare. Scoring of the ACA anticipates $390 billion in Medicare savings through 2019.[46] The law will also bring in additional payroll tax revenue through the 0.9 percent increase in the Medicare payroll tax, and the imposition of the tax to capital gains and interest and dividend income. That money is funneled through the Medicare Trust Fund.[47]

Government trust fund accounting methodology counts those additional funds as extending the trust fund's solvency and being available to pay future Medicare benefits. But in reality, the funds would be used to purchase special-issue Treasury bonds. When the bonds are purchased, the funds used to purchase them become general revenue and are then spent on the government's annual general operating expenses. What remains behind in the trust fund are the bonds, plus an interest payment attributed to the bonds (also paid in bonds, rather than cash). Government bonds are, in essence, a type of IOU. They are a promise against future tax revenue. When the bonds become due, the government will have to repay them out of general revenue.[48]

In the meantime, however, the government counts on that new general revenue to pay for the cost of the new health legislation. Thus, the government spends the money now, while pretending it is available in the future to pay for future Medicare benefits. That double-counting results in roughly $390 billion. As Medicare's chief actuary points out, "In practice, the improved [Medicare] financing cannot be simultaneously used to finance other Federal outlays (such as the coverage expansions) and to extend the trust fund, despite the appearance of this result from the respective accounting conventions."[49]

The same is true regarding $53 billion in additional Social Security taxes generated under the ACA. The CBO assumes that, as discussed earlier, many employers may ultimately decide that it is cheaper to "pay than play" and will stop offering health insurance to their workers. The CBO assumes that in those cases, workers will receive higher wages to offset at least some of the loss in nonwage (insurance) compensation. However, the workers will have to pay taxes, including Social Security payroll taxes, on those additional wages. The additional revenue from those taxes is counted in the CBO's scoring of the ACA. Because they are paying additional taxes, those workers are also accruing additional Social Security benefits, and as those benefits will be paid outside the 10-year budget window, the cost of the additional benefits is not included in the scoring. Only one side of the revenue–benefit equation is included.

When all additional costs are included, the ACA's real 10-year cost appears to be much closer to $2.63 trillion. Since the legislation includes roughly $1.33 trillion in new or increased taxes through 2024 to pay for the benefits it provides, a calculation of the law's full costs suggests it will add $1.3 trillion to the national debt over that period.[50]

Figure 8.3
ACA OUTLAYS AND REVENUES THROUGH 2024

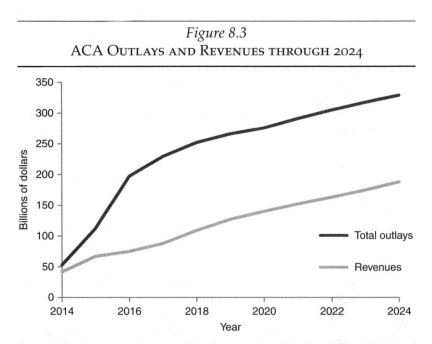

SOURCE: Author's calculations using Congressional Budget Office, "Updated Estimates of the Effects on Health Insurance and the Federal Budget for the Insurance Coverage Provisions in the Affordable Care Act—April 2014," April 14, 2014; Congressional Budget Office, Letter from Douglas W. Elmendorf, director, Congressional Budget Office, to the Honorable John Boehner on H.R. 6079, July 24, 2012.

Moreover, as figure 8.3 shows, the cost trajectory at the end of the 10-year budget window is headed higher. Thus, we can anticipate even higher costs, additional taxes, and an added debt burden in the out years.

One important caveat: all of these estimates are based on currently projected levels of subsidies. If, as noted above, the Supreme Court rules that federally run exchanges cannot offer subsidies, the program's cost would decline significantly—pending a Congressional response of course.

Paying the Bill

To pay for everything, the ACA imposes roughly $1.33 trillion in new or increased taxes through 2024. Depending on exactly how one defines a "tax," the ACA imposes or increases roughly 19 separate taxes, falling on both businesses and individuals.[51] They include the following:

- **Tax on "Cadillac" insurance plans**. One of the most heavily debated new taxes in the health care bill was the tax on high-cost insurance plans. Beginning in 2018, a 40 percent excise tax will be imposed on employer-provided insurance plans with an actuarial value in excess of $10,200 for an individual or $27,500 for families. (The threshold is increased to $11,850 for individuals and $30,950 for families whose head of household is over the age of 55 or engaged in high-risk professions, such as police officers, firefighters, or miners.) The tax falls on the value of the plan over the threshold and is paid by the insurer, or the employer if self-insured.[52] The benefit value of employer-sponsored coverage would include the value of contributions to employees' flexible spending, health reimbursement, and health savings accounts. It is estimated that 12 percent of workers will initially have policies that are subject to the tax.[53] However, the tax is indexed to inflation rather than the faster-rising medical inflation, which drives insurance premiums. As a result, more and more workers will eventually find their insurance plans falling subject to the tax. In fact, a study for the benefits consulting firm Towers Watson concludes, "Assuming even reasonable annual plan cost increases to project 2018 costs, many of today's average plans will easily exceed the cost ceilings directed at today's 'gold-plated' plans."[54]

- **Payroll tax hike**. The Medicare payroll tax was increased from 2.9 percent today to 3.8 percent for individuals with incomes over $200,000 for a single individual or $250,000 for a couple.[55] The payroll tax hike would mean that in eight states, workers would face marginal tax rates in excess of 50 percent.

- **Tax on investment income**. Starting in 2013, the 3.8 percent Medicare tax was applied to capital gains and interest and dividend income if an individual's total gross income exceeds $200,000 or a couple's income exceeds $250,000.[56] The tax applies only to the amount of income in excess of those limits but would be based on total income. Thus, if a couple had $200,000 in wage income and $100,000 in capital gains, $50,000 would be taxed. Moreover, the definition of "capital gains" includes capital gains from the sale of real estate, meaning that an individual who sold his or her home for a profit of $200,000 or more would be subject to the tax. Given the current weakness in the housing market, that tax burden would seem to create a particularly pernicious outcome. Numerous studies have shown that high capital gains taxes discourage investment, resulting in lower economic growth, fewer jobs, and reduced wages.

- **Limit on itemized deductions.** Beginning in 2013, the threshold at which taxpayers can deduct medical expenses was raised from 7.5 percent of adjusted gross income to a new floor of 10 percent.[57] The increased threshold is postponed until 2016 for taxpayers age 65 or older.[58]

- **Tax on prescription drugs**. The legislation imposes a new tax on brand-name prescription drugs designed to raise a specific amount of money annually. Rather than imposing a specific tax amount, the legislation identifies a specific amount of revenue to be raised, ranging from $2.5 billion in 2011 to $4.2 billion in 2018, before leveling off at $2.8 billion thereafter, and assigns a proportion of that amount to pharmaceutical manufacturers according to a formula based on the company's aggregate revenue from branded prescription drugs.[59] The structure of this tax almost guarantees that it will be passed along to consumers through higher prices.

- **Tax on medical devices**. A 2.3 percent federal sales tax is imposed on medical devices, which include everything from CT scanners to surgical scissors.[60] The secretary of HHS has the authority to waive this tax for items that are "sold at retail for use by the general public."[61] However, almost everything used by doctors, hospitals, or clinics would be taxed. The tax would also fall on laboratory tests. The government's chief actuary has concluded that this tax, as with those on pharmaceutical manufacturers and insurers "would generally be passed through to health consumers."[62] In fact, a study by the Republican staff of the Joint Economic Committee estimates that the pass-through could cost the typical family of four with job-based coverage an additional $1,000 a year in higher premiums.[63]

- **Additional taxes on insurers**. Similar to the tax on pharmaceutical companies, the legislation imposes a tax on health insurers based on their market share.[64] The total assessment will begin at $8 billion and rise to $14.3 billion by 2018. Thereafter the total assessment will increase by the same percentage as premium growth for the previous year.[65] The tax will be allocated according to a formula based on both the total premiums collected by an insurer and the insurer's administrative costs.[66] However, some insurers in Michigan and Nebraska received a special exemption.[67] This tax is also expected to be passed through to consumers through higher premiums. (Interestingly, AARP is exempt from this tax on sales of its highly profitable Medigap policies.)[68]

The combination of taxes and subsidies in the ACA results in a substantial redistribution of income. The new law will cost families earning more than $348,000 per year (top 1 percent of incomes) an additional $52,000 per year on average in new taxes and reduced benefits.[69] In contrast, those earning $18,000–$55,000 per year will see a net income increase of roughly $2,000 per family.[70]

The CBO projects that revenue raised from those taxes will more than offset the cost of the program, resulting in a deficit reduction of $109 billion through 2022.[71] However, as we saw earlier, the CBO underestimates the actual cost of the ACA. If we use a more accurate accounting of the program's full cost, the ACA could add as much as $1.4 trillion in additional debt over 10 years, and far more in the years outside the budget window.

It could—and likely will—be even worse than that, because the ACA will almost certainly slow economic growth, thereby reducing revenues.

Take the effect on jobs, for instance. As discussed earlier, the ACA requires businesses with 50 or more full-time employees to provide health insurance coverage to their workers or pay a penalty. That magic number of 50 becomes extremely important, since companies with fewer than 50 workers are not subject to the mandate; that is, they suffer no penalty for not providing insurance to their workers. Suppose, therefore, that a firm with 49 employees does not provide health benefits. Hiring one more worker will trigger a penalty of $2,000 per worker multiplied by the entire workforce, after subtracting the statutory exemption for the first 30 workers. If you were that small-business owner with 49 employees, how fast would you run out to hire that 50th worker? (In France, another country where numerous government regulations kick in at 50 workers, there were 1,500 companies with 48 employees and 1,600 with 49 employees in 2011, but just 660 with 50 and only 500 with 51.)[72]

In fact, according to a Gallup poll conducted in the summer of 2013, 41 percent of small businesses said they have already held off on plans to hire new employees, and 38 percent said they've pulled back on plans to expand their businesses in other ways.[73] Another survey, conducted by the U.S. Chamber of Commerce and the International Franchise Association, of businesses just above the 50-employee threshold found that 59 percent of franchises and 52 percent of non-franchises say that they will "make personnel changes to stay below the 50 full time equivalent employee threshold."[74]

In addition to laying off workers, some companies appear to be trying to reduce the number of employees subject to the mandate either by reducing the number of current employees to fewer than 50 or by shifting full-time workers to part-time, for whom the mandate doesn't apply. According to Gallup, 19 percent of small businesses indicate that they have already laid off workers, and a similar proportion indicated they had cut back their hours.[75]

Even more significant, numerous companies have reportedly reduced the work hours of some employees to keep them below the 30-hour ceiling that would define them as "full-time" for purposes of the mandate. Ben Casselman, writing for FiveThirtyEight, finds that the percent of part-time workers working 25 to 29 hours increased from 9.7 percent before the law passed to 11.1 percent in 2013. Over the same period, the percentage of workers with hours just above the threshold, 31 to 34 hours a week, fell from 7.7 percent to 6.6 percent.[76] While he stresses that it is difficult to disentangle how much of this decline can be attributed to Obamacare, "the timing is suggestive: The change in working hours appears to hit in the middle of 2013, as the major components of the law were beginning to take effect."[77]

Even companies well above the 50-employee cutoff will be affected. Nearly all economists agree that the amount of compensation each worker receives is a function of his or her productivity, and the employer is indifferent to the makeup of that compensation among wages, taxes, insurance premiums, or other costs associated with that worker's employment. Mandating an increase in a worker's compensation (through the provision of health insurance) increases the worker's operating costs without increasing the worker's productivity.

Roughly 96 percent of those companies offer health insurance today.[78] But, as discussed earlier, the ACA may drive up the cost of that insurance, both through general premium hikes and by requiring companies to offer a more expansive and expensive benefits package. Either way, employers must find ways to offset the added costs imposed by the mandate. Whether they do it by reducing wages and benefits, increasing prices, or reducing employment, the effect on the economy will be negative.

Nor should we ignore the impact of the taxes that the ACA imposes on businesses. The 2.3 percent gross income tax on medical device manufacturers alone is estimated to put as many as 43,000 jobs at risk.[79] A tax on insurers is projected to jeopardize another 125,000 to 249,000 jobs, according to the National Federation of Independent Business.[80] The effect of other taxes is harder to specify, but by raising taxes on capital, for example, the ACA will reduce the availability of funding for future investment.[81]

Moreover, it's not just the direct cost of the taxes that will burden businesses. It is estimated that businesses will have to spend at least 127.6 million hours complying with the law.[82] Those hours represent a significant loss of productive manpower.

Chris Conover of the Center for Health Policy and Inequalities Research at Duke University estimates that the ACA's tax and regulatory burdens will reduce economic growth in this country by $157 billion to $550 billion over the next decade and will kill 1,139,000 to 1,625,000 jobs.[83]

The availability of subsidies may also induce some workers to quit their jobs voluntarily, especially older workers seeking early retirement. The CBO recently warned that because of the law, the equivalent of 2.5 million full-time workers will leave the labor force over the next 10 years.[84] Although that may well be good news for those workers who are now able to retire earlier than they otherwise would have—and to be free, in House Minority Leader Nancy Pelosi's memorable phrase "to write poetry"—the loss of those workers, many at the peak of their productivity, will hurt the economy as a whole. According to the CBO, it will reduce aggregate labor compensation by 1 percent over the period 2017–2024, twice the initial estimate.[85]

Finally, we should recognize that the ACA will increase the overall size of government and the share of the economy taken up by government spending. As we saw in Chapter 1, that growth in government is, in itself, a drag on economic growth.

As a result, the ACA's taxes will almost certainly bring in less revenue than projected, meaning deficits and debt will be higher. That growing debt will further depress growth, leading to a cycle of economic decline.

The Impact of Rising Premiums

The ACA's impact on insurance premiums is a highly complex issue that does not lend itself to the easy analysis suggested by some observers on both the left (lower premiums) and right (higher premiums). In reality, 2014 premiums were probably lower for some consumers (especially after fully accounting for subsidies), and higher for others. A study by Avik Roy of the Manhattan Institute compared premiums for policies available through exchanges with the average cost of the five least expensive pre-ACA plans for the most populous zip code in every county, after adjusting for the denial and surcharge rates of those plans, which increase the effective premium amount.

He analyzed premium increases for three ages: 27, 40, and 64. The ACA's effect on premiums varies by age group, but overall the average state will face underlying premium increases of 41 percent. [86]

Still, one bit of good news for ACA costs is the fact that, overall, exchange-based premiums appear to be lower than previous projections from the CBO.[87] (Or more accurately, premiums are lower than CBO-projected premiums for 2016, reverse-engineered to provide a 2013 estimate.)[88] Lower premiums mean lower subsidy costs.

Of course, one should be careful about projecting a trend from one year's premiums. Premiums in 2015 saw modest increases on average, but some of the most popular plans saw more significant premium hikes. In roughly a fifth of the counties in states using the federal insurance exchange, premiums for the lowest-priced silver plans will increase by 10 percent or more. At the same time, premiums for comparable plans will decrease in all of Maine, Montana, and New Hampshire.[89] An analysis by the Kaiser Family Foundation looked at the benchmark Silver and Bronze plans in every county (which account for the majority of enrollees). Across all counties, the Bronze plans saw a four percent increase and Silver plans two percent, but there was a wide degree of variation among states. Alaska's Silver plan premiums increased by 26.5 percent and Mississippi's decreased by 25.5 percent.[90]

There is also reason to believe that premium hikes in future years could be even larger. Since Obamacare depends on overcharging the young and healthy to subsidize the older and sicker, it needs roughly 40 percent of enrollees to be in the 18–34 age group. We don't yet know the health status of those signing up, although evidence from pharmaceutical-purchase patterns analyzed by Express Scripts suggests that enrollees are less healthy than the population at large.[91] Preliminary surveys of self-reported health status seem to corroborate those findings. For example, a Gallup survey found that just 37 percent of exchange enrollees reported they were in excellent or very good health, compared with 50 percent of the population at large.[92]

Meanwhile, we do know that just 28 percent of those signing up during the first year of open enrollment were 18 to 34, meaning that Obamacare missed its target by almost a third.[93] Some states missed by even more. Only 20 percent of those enrolling in Hawaii were "young invincibles," and just 21 percent were in Arizona.[94] Through the first month of the 2015 open enrollment period, only 24 percent were in this 18 to 34 group, which could further skew the risk pools.[95]

The result of such "adverse selection" is that the pool of insured Americans will be much less healthy than predicted, meaning that it will cost more than estimated to provide them with benefits. By and large, young people are healthier and use less health care than do those who are older. For example, only 2.7 percent of those 18 to 34 rate themselves in "fair" or "poor" health, whereas 5.3 percent of those ages 35 to 50 and 9.6 percent of those ages 51 to 64 do so.[96] Those 18- to 34-year-olds see a doctor only 2.7 times per year on average, but 35- to 50-year-olds average 3.3 physician visits per year and 51- to 64-year-olds average 4.8.[97]

If the insurance pool is composed largely of people who are older and sicker, and who therefore use more and more expensive health care, insurance prices will rise to cover their costs. That rate increase will then cause even more young and healthy people to drop their insurance, leaving the pools even older and sicker than before. That raises premiums yet again, leading to the healthiest remaining participants to drop out, and so on. Actuaries refer to that result as the "adverse-selection death spiral."

In the meantime, subsidies will have to increase in order to offset the rising premiums. In addition, the government may have to bail out the insurance companies, providing them with subsidies, in order to prevent the death spiral. Taxpayers pick up the tab for 78 percent of claim costs between $45,000 and $250,000 per insured individual.[98]

It seems safe to say, therefore, that if premiums rise in the future, so will the cost of Obamacare. Thus, we have one more reason to assume that the ACA will ultimately cost more than predicted.

Bang for the Buck?

As we can see, the ACA will be extraordinarily costly. But adding insult to injury, it will fall far short of its stated goal of providing all Americans with access to quality, affordable health insurance.[99]

In fact, even if the ACA worked precisely as its authors intended, it would not come close to universal coverage. At the time the law passed, the CBO estimated that roughly 32 million uninsured Americans would either be covered through Medicaid or private insurance, leaving some 23 million uninsured.[100] Since then, each successive estimate reduced the number of people who would gain coverage. The most recent estimates suggest that as few as 26 million out of the 57 million who would be uninsured in 2024 would eventually be covered as a result of the ACA.[101] Roughly 13 million of those would be enrolled in Medicaid, meaning just 12 million to 13 million previously uninsured would receive private insurance coverage.[102]

So far, the program's participation rates suggest that there is reason to wonder whether or not it will meet even that limited goal.

It is true that the most recent poll from Gallup found that the uninsured rate fell to 12.9 percent in the fourth quarter of 2014, down from 16.3 percent before the ACA was passed.

Of course, it would be a mistake to attribute all of that improvement to the ACA. A large portion may be due to falling unemployment as the economy finally emerges from the recession. Since most Americans get their health insurance through their jobs, lower unemployment should naturally reduce the number of uninsured. Still, the ACA can rightly be credited with some of the gains.

As of the time this book went to press it was estimated that roughly 9 million Americans will have enrolled in health insurance plans through an exchange during the ACA's first two years of operation.[103] That does represent a significant achievement, especially given the troubles that accompanied the initial rollout of healthcare.gov. That may slightly overstate actual enrollment numbers, however, since not every "enrollee" will actually follow through and pay the premiums.

Moreover, 8 million enrollees doesn't necessarily mean 8 million more Americans with insurance. For starters, as many as 6 million Americans had to change their health plans because Obamacare banned the policy they'd had before (see next section). Many of those whose plans got canceled bought new insurance through the exchanges, and are among the 8 million. How many? Estimates vary, but a recent survey by The Commonwealth Fund estimates that 59 percent of exchange enrollees were previously insured.[104]

It is also estimated that roughly 6.4 million Americans have received Medicaid coverage as a result of the ACA (although there may be methodological problems with this estimate).[105] However, as noted in Chapter 7, Medicaid coverage does not necessarily mean better access to care. It is also possible that a substantial number of Medicaid enrollees may have dropped private insurance in order to obtain Medicaid.[106] These Medicaid enrollees may actually now be receiving worse care than they had before.

Finally, estimates suggest that the ACA enabled roughly 1 million young people to stay on their parents' insurance policies. (The administration's often cited estimate of 3 million young people being able to stay on their parents' policy is a result of cherry-picking the numbers.)

Putting it all together, the ACA may have succeeded in covering about 23 percent of the 55 million Americans who were uninsured in 2013. In fact, the CBO projects that for Obamacare to reach its intended targets, exchange enrollment will have to more than triple by 2016.[107] That seems like a pretty tall order.

Other Problems with the ACA

Any discussion of the costs of the ACA would be remiss without at least a mention of the many other problems facing the program.

You Probably Can't Keep Your Current Insurance

One thing we now know for sure is that President Obama's promise that "if you like your health-care plan, you'll be able to keep your health-care plan, period"[108]—a promise he repeated at least 30 times—has, in the president's own words, "ended up not being accurate."[109]

As of December 2013, roughly 5.4 million Americans with individual policies have had their current insurance cancelled because it did not meet the ACA's requirements.[110] Another 3 million to 8 million are expected to lose their policies in the coming months.[111]

The president has made the point that that estimate is only "a small amount of the population."[112] He is correct that, the individual insurance market, in which most cancellations have occurred so far, represents only about 5 percent of Americans. However, it is only the tip of the iceberg.

Because the president has postponed the employer mandate, the 55 percent of Americans who receive their insurance through work have seen far fewer cancellations than people in the individual market (except in cases where employers have dropped coverage; see below). But the same ACA provisions that have resulted in the cancellation of individual policies will start to affect employer-sponsored plans by late 2014.

Why all those cancellations? In essence, the problem starts with the law's mandates themselves. As already noted, if the government is going to require you to buy or provide insurance, then it must define what is and is not insurance. To satisfy the mandate, insurance must meet certain government-defined standards for "minimum essential coverage."[113] If you have insurance, but it does not meet those standards, you cannot continue with that plan, even "if you like your plan."

Individuals and businesses that had insurance prior to March 31, 2010, are "grandfathered in," meaning they theoretically do not have to change their current insurance to meet the new minimum benefit requirements.[114] However, if any "substantial change" was made to the plan after March 2010, or if any such change is made in the future, the plan loses its grandfathered status and can no longer be sold by the insurer. It does not matter whether those changes are (were) instigated by the individual or by the insurer. If there is a substantial change, the plan must change in order to comply with the ACA requirements.

The ACA did not specify what would be considered a "substantial change," but HHS subsequently issued regulations defining substantial change as (a) significantly cutting or reducing benefits, (b) raising copays by more than $5 (or the rate of medical inflation), (c) increasing deductibles over a certain threshold, (d) lowering employer contributions, and (e) raising coinsurance charges.[115]

As a result, millions of current plans in the individual market have lost their grandfathered status. (The group or employer market will be discussed later). And since many of those plans did not meet ACA requirements, those plans are being cancelled.

The president attempted to reduce the number of cancellations by allowing insurers, if they wished, to reinstate noncompliant plans for one year, if state insurance commissioners agreed.[116] However, that transition policy was much more difficult to carry out in practice than the presidential directive indicated.

Insurance plans are not simply a list of benefits on a piece of paper. They are a complex interrelationship between benefits, the pool of insured customers, a network of providers, and so on. And because insurers had been told for three years that they could not sell noncompliant plans, many of those plans simply didn't exist anymore. Even where they could be re-created, it requires a time-consuming and costly process. Moreover, many of those who have had their plans cancelled have already bought new policies, sometimes with different insurers. As a result, insurers have been reluctant to go along.

State insurance commissioners were also less than receptive. Commissioners in 11 states and the District of Columbia have refused to allow insurers to reinstate noncompliant plans. They include many of the states with the largest number of cancellations, such as California and New York.[117] To date, no accurate tally exits of how many plans were ultimately reinstated. But the anecdotal evidence suggests that very few have been.

This "cancellation fix" was originally supposed to be for only one year, but the extension will now allow people to renew such plans until 2016, with coverage lasting in some cases until September 2017, depending on when exactly customers renew their plans.[118] That extension significantly increases the uncertainty insurers face when trying to set premium rates in the next few years, which could make rate shocks more likely.

Some have argued that the only plans affected were exceptionally skimpy plans that failed to provide basic health care benefits, "crappy" plans in the words of one Obama administration official, or "subpar," as the president put it.[119] The *New York Times* even wrongly suggested that the plans being cancelled failed to cover some basic benefits like hospitalization.[120]

No doubt, some individual plans *were* less than comprehensive. However, most plans failed ACA compliance for relatively minor reasons. According to HealthPocket, a health insurance consulting firm, fewer than 2 percent of individual policies in place in 2013 met all ACA requirements.[121] The most frequent reason for noncompliance was not a failure to cover hospitalization but a lack of pediatric care, including vision and dental care for children. Just 24 percent of individual plans provided that benefit.[122] But for childless individuals, it's hard to see the lack of such a benefit rendering the policy "subpar."

The other frequently missing benefits included maternity and newborn care (not included in 64 percent of plans), drug and alcohol rehabilitation (46 percent), and mental health benefits (39 percent).[123] There may indeed be reasons, such as enlarging risk pools and cross subsidization, for wanting men or those beyond childbearing age to purchase maternity care, for nondrinkers to purchase alcohol rehabilitation, and so on; but that is far different from claiming that those plans do not offer adequate benefits to the purchasers themselves.

As noted, so far nearly all of the cancelled policies have been individual plans, a relatively small part of the insurance market. Most Americans receive their insurance through their job. What will happen to them? Employer plans change frequently today. Most of those changes are relatively minor, and employees may not even notice the difference. In a technical sense, it could be said that they are not keeping their current insurance plan today. However the ACA will expand and accelerate this process, and the change in insurance for many employees will become far more significant.

As previously noted, under the ACA, group insurance sold through the employer market is subject to the same requirements as individual insurance. However, large numbers of employer plans do not fully meet those requirements.

As with individual policies, plans that were in place before March 2010 are "grandfathered," so long as there is no substantial change in the plan.[124] However, because company plans frequently undergo routine changes, barely a third of covered workers are in grandfathered employer-sponsored plans. Interestingly, small businesses, which have been aggressively trying to "lock in" their current plans, are more likely to be grandfathered than are larger employers. A bit more than half of the businesses with 50 or fewer workers have a grandfathered plan, whereas only 30 percent of companies with more than 5,000 employees offer one.[125]

The mix of grandfathered and noncompliant plans varies and does not perfectly overlap. Smaller firms are more likely to offer noncompliant plans but be grandfathered. Larger companies may not be grandfathered but are more likely to be compliant. Overall, according to Avik Roy of the Manhattan Institute, roughly half of the employer-based insurance market is currently neither grandfathered nor compliant.[126] Given the frequency with which companies make changes to their plans, as already noted, few companies will maintain their grandfathering over the long run.[127] In 2011, the Congressional Research Service estimated that, because of those restrictions, 66 percent of small-employer plans and 51 percent of all plans will lose grandfathered status by the end of 2013.[128]

At the time the ACA was enacted, HHS estimated that 66 percent of small businesses and 45 percent of larger businesses would eventually have to change their plans.[129] That would mean as many as 78 million workers could lose their current employer-provided plan.[130]

Unlike with individual policies, no comprehensive survey data are available to show exactly where existing employer plans may fall short of ACA compliance. Still, it seems likely that the majority of noncompliant employer plans suffer from the same noncompliance issues as individual plans. They cover basic insurance benefits but fail to offer one or more of the ACA-specified benefits, such as maternity care or alcohol rehabilitation.

You May Not Be Able to Keep Your Current Doctor

Those who are forced to change their insurance plan may also have to change their doctors. Not every plan includes every doctor in its network. Even a change from one employer-sponsored plan to another may leave workers with a new network that does not include their previous physician.

The problem is more pronounced for those forced to buy a new plan through an exchange. Insurance plans available on the exchanges—and in most states the selection of available plans is extremely limited—have been rapidly dropping doctors and hospitals from their networks. According to a survey by the Medical Group Management Association, nearly 40 percent of doctors are uncertain about whether they will be included in networks of plans being sold through the exchanges.[131] And a new study by PricewaterhouseCoopers warns that "insurers passed over major medical centers" in their California, Illinois, Indiana, Kentucky, and Tennessee networks, among others.[132]

In New York, for example, many exchange-based plans exclude the Memorial Sloan Kettering Cancer Center, widely regarded as one of the world's premier cancer facilities.[133] In Illinois, Blue Cross and Blue Shield said that at least some of its plans will no longer include Rush University Medical Center or Northwestern Memorial Hospital in their networks.[134] In California, most insurers won't include UCLA Medical Center or Cedars-Sinai. Vanderbilt Hospital is being excluded from many plans in Tennessee.[135] In New Hampshire, Anthem Blue Cross Blue Shield, the only insurer participating in the exchange, covers just 16 of the state's 26 hospitals and has dropped about a third of the physicians who used to be part of its network.[136] Even the Mayo Clinic has been excluded from most plans sold in Minnesota.[137]

In most cases, the decision to exclude providers from a plan has been made by insurers. The ACA's regulations, such as requiring coverage of individuals with preexisting conditions, mandating new benefits, and prohibiting annual or lifetime limits, have driven up costs for insurers. Although insurers have offset some of the increased costs through higher premiums (see below), there are limits to their ability to raise prices, especially for plans sold through exchanges. As a spokesperson for Primera Blue Cross, the dominant insurer in the Seattle area, explained its decision to exclude Seattle Children's Hospital from its network, the hospital's "non-unique services were too expensive given the goal of providing affordable coverage for consumers."[138]

In other cases, the physician or hospital rejects participation in a plan because reimbursement rates are too low. Insurers have been slashing reimbursement rates for plans sold through the exchanges. In some cases, insurers will reimburse physicians and hospitals at levels barely higher than Medicaid. UnitedHealth Group, for example, has cut reimbursements to some New York City doctors to less than $40 for a typical office visit, and about $20 for reading a mammogram.[139] Many physicians and hospitals are likely to decide that participation in the exchange-based plans is just not worth it.

The problem is made worse by the limited choice of insurance plans available through the exchanges (noted earlier). If the only available insurer or insurers decide to exclude your physician or hospital from their networks, an alternative plan may not be available.

Of course, one can always see a physician outside the plan's network. In such cases, insurers generally pay a far lower percentage of the cost. A McKinsey & Company analysis found that 47 percent of the 955 plans available in the first 13 states to make plan filings public were HMOs or similarly designed plans, which usually pay nothing for providers that are not part of their networks.[140] Most other plans were preferred provider organizations, which pay only part of charges for doctors and hospitals outside their networks. In New York, for example, not a single insurance plan offered through the exchange pays anything for out-of-network providers.[141]

The bottom line, as Dr. Ezekiel Emanuel, one of the architects of the ACA and a top adviser to the Obama administration, explained on Fox News, is that you can keep your current doctor "if you want to pay more."[142]

Moreover, if, as some predict, the ACA drives large numbers of physicians out of practice, you could have even more difficulty seeing the physician of your choice. It is, of course, far too early to know how physicians will react in practice, but many appear to be at least open to the possibility of leaving.

The Deloitte 2013 Survey of U.S. Physicians found that 62 percent believe that many physicians will retire and 55 percent believe many will scale back practice hours based on how the future of medicine is changing.[143] A survey by the Physicians Foundation found that roughly half of doctors planned to make changes to their practice that would reduce patient access.[144] In California, the head of the largest medical association in the state estimates that as many as 7 out of 10 physicians could decide not to participate in the state health insurance exchanges, which would dramatically restrict options for exchange enrollees in the state.[145] Of course, not every doctor who told those polls that he or she would consider leaving the field will actually do so. But if even a small percentage departs, our access to medical care will suffer.

For many physicians, retirement in Florida may begin to look like a very good option. More than 47 percent of doctors are age 50 or older.[146] Are they really going to want to stick it out for a few more years if all they have to look forward to is more red tape (both government and insurance company) for less money? Those who remain are increasingly likely to join "concierge practices," limiting the number of patients they see and refusing both government and private insurance. At the same time, fewer young people are likely to decide that medicine is a good career.

Even before the ACA, health care experts estimated that the United States faced a shortage of at least 130,000 physicians, given the needs of a growing and aging population.[147] In fact, we have fewer doctors per capita than such countries as Portugal or Ukraine.[148]

The ACA sets the table for a potential widespread physician shortage. We don't yet know if that will occur or whether, despite their expressed concerns, physicians will ultimately adapt to the changes brought about by the ACA, but there are clearly ominous warning signs.

Consumers May Face Higher Costs

Finally, as previously noted, consumers may see their premiums and other out-of-pocket costs increase significantly.

The preceding discussion focused on the individual market because increases in individual premiums will drive up the cost of subsidies and therefore the ACA's overall cost to taxpayers. But those premium increases will also be a burden to individual consumers as well. The *National Journal* conducted an in-depth independent analysis and concluded that "for the vast majority of Americans, premium prices will be higher in the individual exchange than what they're currently paying," even after accounting for subsidies.[149]

In looking at the cost of insurance, one must also consider out-of-pocket cost sharing, including deductibles, copayments, and coinsurance. Bronze plans, for example, have the lowest premiums of any plans on the exchanges, but they have much higher cost-sharing provisions. Other forms of cost sharing such as copayments and coinsurance could also be quite high.

Notably, the ACA was supposed to cap the total amount of out-of-pocket insurance costs. However, the Department of Labor has delayed the enforcement of those caps for some insurers.[150] Consequently, at least some consumers could face much higher out-of-pocket costs.

Of course, averages are just that. Different groups will be affected differently. In particular, younger and healthier Americans are more likely to see their premiums increase, whereas older and sicker Americans are more likely to find reduced premiums. Indeed, such cross subsidization is fundamental to the design of the ACA.

For employer-sponsored plans, estimates of how the ACA will affect premiums are even harder to come by. At the time the ACA was signed into law, the CBO estimated that premiums would double by 2020. According to the CBO projections, small businesses would see increases roughly in line with that baseline under the ACA, whereas larger businesses could see increases slightly (about 5 percent) below the base line.[151]

More recent studies suggest that premiums for small businesses will actually be higher under the ACA than they would have otherwise been. A recent survey by Milliman, for example, found that small group premiums in the six states analyzed would increase between 6 percent and 12 percent beyond what they would have been in the absence of the ACA.[152] And a report for the House Committee on Energy and Commerce projected increases ranging from 13 percent to 101 percent, based on responses from a limited sample of 17 insurers throughout the country.[153]

Meanwhile, large employers expect their cost of health care benefits to rise almost 4.5 percent in 2014, according to an annual survey conducted by the Kaiser Family Foundation. That comes on top of a similar increase in 2013.[154]

If adverse selection becomes a major problem, future premium increases will likely be much higher, for both individual and employer-sponsored plans.

Although decreased choice, dropped plans, and increased premiums may not show up directly in the federal budget, they are still costs to consumers, patients, workers, and the U.S. economy that should not be ignored.

An Alternative Approach

If the Patient Protection and Affordable Care Act is not the route to health care reform, is there a better way? In short, what would free-market health reform look like?

First, we need to move away from a system dominated by employer-provided health insurance and instead make health insurance personal and portable, controlled by the individual rather than by government or an employer. There is, after all, no logical reason for individuals to receive health insurance through their jobs. We don't, in fact, receive most other types of insurance—auto, homeowners, life—in that way.

Employer-based health insurance is actually an anomaly that grew out of unique historical circumstances during World War II.

Despite the widespread entry of women into the labor force during the war, the shift of men from private employment to the military created a labor shortage. At the same time, wage controls prevented employers from competing for available workers by raising wages. In an effort to circumvent the wage controls and compete for available workers, employers began to offer nonwage benefits, including health insurance. In 1953, the Internal Revenue Service ruled that employer-provided health insurance was *not* part of wage compensation for tax purposes.[155]

Thus, if a worker is paid $40,000, but the employer also provides an insurance policy worth $10,000, the worker pays taxes on just the $40,000 in wages. If, however, instead of providing insurance, the employer gave the worker a $10,000 raise—allowing the worker to purchase his or her own insurance—he or she would have to pay taxes on $50,000. That situation puts workers who buy their own insurance at a significant disadvantage compared with those who receive insurance through work.

Employment-based insurance seriously distorts our health care system in several ways. Most significantly, it hides much of the true cost of health care to consumers, thereby encouraging overconsumption.

Imagine someone shopping for groceries under a situation where someone else has agreed to pay 86 percent of whatever the bill turns out to be. That shopper would almost certainly buy more and more expensive food than he or she would if they were paying the bill themselves. There would be a lot more steak, and a lot less hamburger. The same holds true for health care.

The RAND Health Insurance Experiment, the largest study ever done of consumer health-purchasing behavior, provides ample evidence that consumers purchase more health care if someone else is paying for it. In particular, families with no copayment used 53 percent more hospital services (measured in dollars) and had 63 percent more visits to doctors, drugs, and other services than did the families with the 95 percent copayment. Overall, the total use of medical resources was 58 percent greater for the group with no copayment, despite virtually identical health outcomes. Even smaller copayment rates produced savings. The study found that an individual with no copayment spent 18 percent more on health care than an individual with a 25 percent copayment. Yet with few exceptions, there was little or no difference in outcomes.[156]

More recently, a study by Liran Einav of Stanford University and his colleagues suggests that the prevalence of third-party payment in the United States has nearly doubled the cost of health care in this country. They looked at the U.S. Medicare program for the elderly, essentially the largest insurance program for the elderly, and a program with very low out-of-pocket costs for participants. They found that the program led to a 23 percent increase in total hospital expenditures (for all ages) between 1965 and 1970. Extrapolating from those estimates, they conclude that the overall spread of third-party health insurance between 1950 and 1990 may account for more than 40 percent of the increase in per capita health spending over that period.[157]

Employer-based health insurance also limits consumer choice, because employers get the final say in the type of insurance a worker will receive. The entire controversy over whether corporations should be required to include contraceptive coverage in their insurance plans is the result of a system in which insurance is based on one's place of employment.[158] A woman who wants an insurance plan covering contraceptives should be able to take the money that the company is currently paying for insurance and buy the policy that she wants, rather than a plan provided by the employer. The worker gets the coverage she wants, and the company doesn't have to directly pay for contraceptive coverage that it is morally opposed to. Everyone wins.

Moreover, our current employment-based health insurance system means that people who don't receive insurance through work are put at a significant and costly disadvantage. And of course, it means that if you lose your job, you are likely to end up uninsured.

Changing from employer to individual insurance requires changing the tax treatment of health insurance. Employer-provided insurance should be treated the same as other compensation for tax purposes: that is, as taxable income. To offset the increased tax, workers should receive a standard deduction, a tax credit, or better still "large health savings accounts" to purchase health insurance, regardless of whether they receive it through their job or purchase it on their own.[159]

As a result of that shift in tax policy, employers would likely gradually begin to substitute higher wages for insurance, allowing the worker to shop for the insurance policy that most closely matched his or her needs. That insurance would more likely be true insurance, protecting the worker against catastrophic risk, while requiring out-of-pocket payment for routine, low-dollar costs, and it would belong to the worker not the employer, meaning that workers would be able to take it from job to job and would not lose it if they became unemployed.

Putting purchasing power in the hands of consumers is only half of market-based reform. The other part of effective health care reform involves increasing competition among both insurers and health providers. Current regulations establish monopolies and cartels in both industries. Today, for example, people can't purchase health insurance across state lines. And because different states have very different regulations and mandates, costs can vary widely depending on where you live.

New Jersey, for example, requires insurers to cover a wide range of procedures and types of care, including in vitro fertilization, contraceptives, and chiropodists, and coverage of children until they reach age 25. Those mandated benefits aren't cheap. According to a 2006 analysis by the National Center for Policy Analysis, the cost of a standard health insurance policy for a healthy 25-year-old man averaged $5,580 in the state. A standard policy in Kentucky, which has far fewer mandates, would cost the same man only $960 per year.[160]

Unfortunately, consumers are more or less held prisoner by their state's regulatory regime. It is illegal for that hypothetical New Jersey resident to buy the cheaper health insurance in Kentucky. On the other hand, if consumers were free to purchase insurance in other states, they could in effect "purchase" the regulations of that other state. Consumers in New Jersey could avoid the state's regulatory costs and choose, say, Kentucky, if that state's regulations aligned more closely with their preferences.

With millions of American consumers balancing costs and risks, states would be forced to evaluate whether their regulations offered true value or simply reflected the influence of special interests.

We also need to rethink medical-licensing laws to encourage greater competition among providers. Nurse practitioners, physician assistants, midwives, and other nonphysician practitioners should have far greater ability to treat patients.[161] We should also be encouraging such innovations in delivery as medical clinics in retail outlets.

A Costly New Program

Whatever one thinks of the goals of the Affordable Care Act, it will no doubt add significantly to the burden facing this country's finances. Although we were once promised that health care reform would "bend the cost curve down,"[162] the law will actually *increase* U.S. health care spending. That failure to control costs means that the law will add significantly to the already-crushing burden of government spending, taxes, and debt. Accurately measured, the Patient Protection and Affordable Care Act will cost more than $2.6 trillion over the next 10 years and will add more than $1.3 trillion to the national debt.

The ACA will also significantly burden businesses, thereby posing a substantial threat to economic growth and job creation. Some businesses may respond to the law's employer mandate by choosing to pay the penalty and dumping their workers into public programs, but many others will be forced to offset increased costs by reducing wages, benefits, or employment.

The legislation also imposes more than $1.3 trillion in new or increased taxes, the vast majority of which will fall on businesses. Many of those taxes, especially those on hospitals, insurers, and medical device manufacturers, will ultimately be passed along through higher health care costs. However, other taxes, in particular new taxes on investment income, will likely reduce economic and job growth. Businesses will also face new administrative and record-keeping requirements under this legislation that will also increase their operating costs, reducing their ability to hire, expand, or increase compensation.

It is also becoming increasingly clear that millions of Americans will not be able to keep their current coverage. While the final bill grandfathered current plans, the reality is that Americans will still be forced to change coverage to a plan that meets government requirements, if there have been any changes since 2010. And, by forbidding noncompliant plans from enrolling any new customers, the law makes those plans nonviable over the long term. Already somewhere in the range of 6 million Americans with individual coverage have been forced to change plans. And, when the employer mandate finally takes full effect, millions more will have to do likewise.

All of this represents an enormous price to pay in exchange for the law's small increases in insurance coverage. There is very little "bang for the buck."

9. Running Out of Other People's Money

A fundamental truism: things that cannot continue forever eventually stop. Or as Margaret Thatcher reputedly said about the problem facing modern welfare states, eventually they "always run out of other people's money."[1]

Today, our national debt is roughly $18 trillion. Let's put that in perspective: The New York Yankees have one of the biggest payrolls in baseball. For $18 trillion, one could pay the 2014 Yankees for 86,335 years and still have money left over for a couple of free-agent pitchers. And speaking of New York, $18 trillion could buy all the real estate in New York City—almost 20 times over. If 18 trillion one-dollar bills were stacked on a football field, they would cover the field to a depth of more than two miles. Alternatively, a single stack of 18 trillion one-dollar bills would be 1.2 million miles high, enough for a round-trip to the moon, twice over. If we were to repay our national debt at the rate of $1 per second, we could wipe it out in a mere 573,400 years.

Beginning to get the idea? We are talking about a lot of money. Each American's share of that debt is nearly $56,496.

But as bad as that sounds, the real situation is actually worse. Our official national debt numbers do not include the unfunded future liabilities for entitlement programs such as Social Security and Medicare. Even under the most optimistic projections, those liabilities, the difference between projected benefits and revenue, total more than $72.5 trillion. Other projections suggest that they could run to more than $130 trillion. Thus, our true total debt is actually somewhere between $90.5 trillion and $130 trillion. That's a debt of at least $282,662 for every man, woman, and child in this country. And it potentially could be as much as $406,034 per person. Students getting out of college today worry about their college debt. That's nothing compared with what they owe as their share of the national debt.[2]

It's true that annual budget deficits have fallen to their lowest level since 2008. The annual deficit is projected to be as little as $469 billion this year. Of course, that still means that we are borrowing almost 15 cents out of every dollar we spend. Even so, tax revenues are up, at their highest levels as a percentage of gross domestic product (GDP) since 2007, and spending, in part thanks to the much-reviled sequester, has fallen to its lowest level, as a percentage of GDP, since 2008.

But that phenomenon is just temporary. According to the Congressional Budget Office (CBO), deficits will start rising as soon as 2016, and by 2024 will approach $1 trillion per year. The CBO also estimates that we will add another $8.8 trillion to the debt through 2024, at which point gross federal debt will be more than $26.5 trillion. At the same time, federal government spending is on track to reach more than 36 percent of GDP by mid–century, and with total federal and state government spending exceeding half of GDP.[3]

Clearly, we are on a course that cannot continue. The question isn't will it stop, but how. Will we find our way to a soft landing that minimizes disruption, allows for renewed economic growth, and protects those Americans who are most vulnerable? Or are we on the road for the turmoil and economic stagnation that we see in countries like Greece? Despite the undeniable fiscal facts, politicians from both parties continue to obfuscate and dodge the difficult decisions that will determine which of those two paths we follow.

Democrats either deny that there is a problem or insist that the problem could be solved if only the wealthy paid higher taxes. But even if one thought that tax increases were a good idea, and could be implemented without killing jobs or slowing economic growth, it is simply impossible to increase taxes enough to close the budget gap. In particular, raising taxes on the wealthy falls far short of what would be required to pay for our current and future obligations.[4]

Besides, much of the current talk about raising taxes seems more about scoring political points than about revenue. The actual tax increases that Democrats have proposed raise hardly any money. For example, President Obama has repeatedly called for closing "high-income tax loopholes," but even his own budget proposal estimates that doing so would only bring in $60 billon through 2024.[5]

Meanwhile, Republicans give frequent lip service to the debt crisis but pretend that you can deal with the debt crisis by eliminating "waste, fraud, and abuse" in the federal budget. Certainly, there is plenty of that, but you simply cannot balance the budget by cutting the usual suspects. Foreign aid amounts to less than 1 percent of federal spending.[6] Federal subsidies to Planned Parenthood and the Corporation for Public Broadcasting amount to a combined 0.02 percent.[7]

In fact, as President Obama proudly, and correctly, points out, even in his bloated budget, domestic discretionary spending will amount to just 2.5 percent of GDP by 2023, a historic low.[8] That is not to say we shouldn't cut those programs. Many are indeed wasteful. Some do more harm than good. Most would probably be better left to the private sector and civil society. Every dollar in savings is a good thing, but the sad fact remains that such cuts come nowhere near balancing the budget or significantly reducing the debt.

Moreover, both Democrats and Republicans appear to have taken our temporary success in reducing the deficit as an excuse to resume taxing and spending. President Obama's FY2016 budget proposals, for instance, would abandon the sequester budget caps. He would increase domestic discretionary spending by $34 billion above those caps next year, while also hiking defense spending by an equal amount.[9] That would amount to a year-over-year discretionary spending increase of 7 percent, compared to an average of 4 percent from 2004–2013.[10]

The president would theoretically pay for this spending spree with a $320 billion tax hike on capital gains, banks' assets, and financial transactions, partially offset by $175 billion in tax cuts targeted to the middle class. Even so, the president's proposals would increase both the deficit and debt projections cited throughout this book.

As of press time, the Republicans had not yet introduced their FY2016 budget plan. But, if their FY2015 budget proposal serves as a guide, we should expect it to be better, but only marginally. The 2015 Republican budget (which, it should be noted, was not actually enacted) did eventually balance the budget, although not until 2024. It would have added another $2.4 trillion to the debt by 2025.[11]

As for FY2016, several Republicans, especially defense hawks such as Senators John McCain (AZ) and Lindsey Graham (SC), have called for eliminating sequester caps for military spending and seem willing to agree to domestic spending hikes as a trade-off.[12]

Advocates of reducing the debt should obviously stand strong against such spending hikes. Still, the simple truth is that there is no way to address America's debt problem without reforming entitlements, notably Social Security, Medicare, Medicaid, and our newest entitlement program, Obamacare.

Social Security, Medicare, and Medicaid alone account for 47 percent of federal spending today, a portion that will only grow larger in the future.[13] And although the spending for Obamacare has just begun, it too will soon consume an ever larger portion of the federal budget. Entitlement spending, not domestic discretionary programs or defense, is where the real money lies.

As we saw in Chapter 5, Social Security will run a $69 billion cash-flow deficit this year. And that's the good news. Every year after, that shortfall will worsen. All together, Social Security is facing future shortfalls worth more than $24.9 trillion.[14] The so-called trust fund is simply an accounting measure, specifying how much money the federal government owes the program out of general revenues, not an actual asset that can be used to pay benefits. At the same time, Social Security taxes are already so high that most young people will receive a rate of return far below historic market returns.

Sadly, Social Security's finances look good compared with those of the government's health care programs.

Medicare, as discussed in Chapter 6, is in even worse financial shape. Depending on how fast health care costs rise, the program's unfunded liabilities could run as high as $89 trillion.[15] Even under the most optimistic scenarios, Medicare's future shortfall approaches $48 trillion.[16] And if savings anticipated under the Affordable Care Act (ACA) fail to materialize, Medicare's long-term costs could be far higher.

Medicaid's financial problems are measured somewhat differently, since the federal portion is funded entirely from general revenues. Nonetheless, the program will cost the federal government almost $300 billion this year, and an additional $150 billion at the state level. Moreover, program costs are rising rapidly. Federal Medicaid costs are estimated to more than double to $576 billion by 2024.[17] After that, as shown in Chapter 7, costs only grow more rapidly.

And if all that was not bad enough, we have now adopted a massive new health care entitlement. The ACA could add $1.3 trillion or more to the deficit over the next 10 years.

We are far beyond the point where "tweaking" those programs—revising them around the edges, cutting a few dollars here, adding a little bit more in taxes there—will forestall the budgetary disaster lurking in our fiscal future.

Moreover, as bad as all those numbers are, it is vital to remember that the debt is merely the most visible symptom of a much bigger issue—the size of government. The federal government currently consumes more than 20.4 percent of GDP.[18] Add in state and local spending, and government consumes more than a third of everything produced in this country. As spending for entitlements rises, government will eventually top 45 percent of GDP.[19] That would be a problem regardless of whether or not the budget was balanced. Indeed, we would likely be better off with an unbalanced federal budget that spent half of what we currently spend.

"Two roads diverged in a yellow wood," wrote Robert Frost, "And sorry I could not travel both."[20] Like Frost's famous traveler, our nation has now reached a fork in the road. Down one path lies business as usual. And although, for the moment, we might see it as straight and easy to pass, it leads to disaster. Following that path means slower economic growth today and a crushing burden of debt for future generations. Take that road and the United States will be Greece.

But there is another path, "the one less traveled by," to extend the metaphor. Taking that route will require our politicians to have the courage to make fundamental, structural reforms to our entitlement programs. That path may appear a bit rocky, because it will mean saying no to powerful interest groups. It will mean looking further into the future than the next election. It will mean recognizing that programs such as Social Security, Medicare, Medicaid, and the ACA not only have become unaffordable but have failed to achieve the goals for which they were created in the first place. But at the end of that path lies renewed prosperity, increased growth, and a brighter future.

It's time to choose a new path. And that, as Frost might say, will make all the difference.

Notes

Chapter 1

1. Congressional Budget Office, "Monthly Budget Review: Summary for Fiscal Year 2014," November 2014; Congressional Budget Office, "Updated Budget Projections: 2014 to 2024," April 2014, http://www.cbo.gov/sites/default/files/cbofiles/attachments/45229-UpdatedBudgetProjections_2.pdf.

2. According to the Treasury Department, $18.08 trillion is the "official" national debt. Department of the Treasury, "Daily Treasury Statement, Thursday, January 8, 2015." It is also the debt most frequently cited by the news media. Accordingly, it is used throughout this book unless otherwise noted. As discussed elsewhere in this chapter, it is derived by combining "debt held by the public" ($12.981 trillion) with "intragovernmental debt" ($5.10 trillion). However, it should be noted that considerable debate exists among economists as to whether that debt figure is the best and most accurate one to use. Many economists would prefer to use only "debt held by the public," sometimes referred to as net debt (with the $18.08 trillion figure referred to as gross debt). Others argue that neither figure accurately reflects the U.S. fiscal balance since neither considers the "asset" side of the ledger, such as the value of federal lands and offshore oil leases. Still others favor generally accepted accounting principles, or some functional equivalent, under which future unfunded liabilities should be fully included. Of course, regardless of which measure is used, the U.S. debt is unacceptably large.

3. Congressional Budget Office, "The 2014 Long-Term Budget Outlook," July 2014, https://www.cbo.gov/sites/default/files/cbofiles/attachments/45308-2014-07-LTBOSuppData_update2.xlsx. Note that this document uses the alternative fiscal scenario for revenue, which projects that revenues will hew to their historical norm of 18.1 percent. Spending data are from the base-line scenario, which could significantly *underestimate* spading levels on entitlements and net interest.

4. Author's calculations based on Congressional Budget Office, "An Update to Budget and Economic Outlook 2014 to 2024: Historical Budget Data," August 2014, https://www.cbo.gov/sites/default/files/cbofiles/attachments/45249-2014-08-HistoricalBudgetData.xlsx.

5. The CBO makes it clear that significant payments from GSEs and TARP were a major component of deficit reduction in 2013 and 2014. In 2013 these two components meant spending was $108 billion lower than it would have otherwise been. In 2014 it was $78 billion. So at least part of what looks like spending restraint is not really attributable to purposeful spending decisions or reductions, but repayment from TARP and Fannie and Freddie. Congressional Budget Office, "Monthly Budget Review: Summary of Fiscal Year 2014."

6. U.S. Census Bureau, "U.S. and World Population Clock," December 31, 2014, http://www.census.gov/popclock.

7. Department of the Treasury, "Daily Treasury Statement, May 28, 2014."

8. Ibid.

9. Ibid.

10. Letter from Douglas Elmendorf, director, Congressional Budget Office, to the Honorable Kent Conrad, August 3, 2010, http://www.cbo.gov/sites/default/files /cbofiles/ftpdocs/117xx/doc11755/08-03-ltbo_letter_conrad.pdf.

11. Government Accountability Office, "Financial Audit: Bureau of the Public Debt's Fiscal Years 2009 and 2008 Schedules of Federal Debt," November 2009, p. 2, https://www.treasurydirect.gov/govt/reports/pd/feddebt/feddebt_ann2009.pdf.

12. Theoretically, one could discount intragovernmental debt as a category and increase the amount of unfunded liabilities. Intragovernmental debt constitutes both an asset to the trust funds and a liability to the federal government as a whole. If one considers general revenues and the various trust funds as a single entity, the debt and asset would simply cancel each other out. However, that does not change the fact that in the future, as payouts from the trust funds are required, the federal government would need to find the money to make those payouts. Since the antici-pated revenue stream falls short of the amount needed to pay those future benefit streams, the expected shortfall would be classified as an unfunded liability or implicit debt. However, the Treasury and others tend to treat intragovernmental debt as being similar to "debt held by the public" since an actual debt instrument (a bond) exists. In the end, that may be a distinction without a difference. Government action could reduce all three types of debt (debt held by the public, intragovernmental debt, and implicit debt), but without action, all three types of debt will eventually come due.

13. That analogy is admittedly imprecise. A portion of the debt—intragovernmen-tal debt—is truly "owed to ourselves" in the sense of being owed by one government entity to another. With credit card debt, the entirety of the debt is owed to an outside entity. However, for purposes of comparison with a family budget, it does represent current accumulated obligations, as opposed to either one-time spending beyond income or future unfunded liabilities.

14. Office of Management and Budget, "Accounting for Liabilities of the Federal Government," Statement of Federal Financial Accounting Standards Number 5, para. 48, September 1995, http://www.fasab.gov/pdffiles/sffas-5.pdf.

15. *The 2014 Annual Report of the Board of Trustees of the Federal Old-Age and Survivors Insurance and Federal Disability Insurance Trust Funds* (Washington: Government Print-ing Office, July 28, 2014), http://www.ssa.gov/oact/tr/2014/tr2014.pdf. This figure does not include the cost of redeeming bonds in the Social Security trust fund, which is properly classified as intergovernmental debt. Some estimates of Social Security's total unfunded liabilities include that intergovernmental debt—since the repayment is unfunded—arriving at a total unfunded liability of more than $27.6 trillion.

16. *2009 Annual Report of the Boards of Trustees of the Federal Hospital Insurance and Federal Supplementary Insurance Trust Funds* (Baltimore: Centers for Medicare and Med-icaid Services, May 12, 2009), https://www.cms.gov/Research-Statistics-Data-and -Systems/Statistics-Trends-and-Reports/ReportsTrustFunds/downloads/tr2009.pdf.

17. *The 2014 Annual Report of the Boards of Trustees of the Federal Hospital Insur-ance and Federal Supplementary Medical Insurance Trust Funds* (Baltimore: Centers for Medicare and Medicaid Services, July 28, 2014), Tables III.BI0, III.C11, III.D7, http:// downloads.cms.gov/files/TR2013.pdf.

18. John Shatto and M. Kent Clemens, "Projected Medicare Expenditures under an Illustrative Scenario with Alternative Payment Updates to Medicare Providers," Office of the Actuary, Centers for Medicare and Medicaid Services, August 5, 2010, http://www.cms.gov/Research-Statistics-Data-and-Systems/Research/ActuarialStudies/downloads/2010TRAlternativeScenario.pdf.

19. Congressional Budget Office, "An Update to Budget Projections: 2014 to 2024."

20. Ibid.

21. Congressional Budget Office, "The 2014 Long-Term Budget Outlook."

22. Author's calculations using information from Federal Reserve Bank of St. Louis, "H.15 Selected Interest Rates: 10-Year Treasury Constant Maturity Rate (DGS10)," http://research.stlouisfed.org/fred2/series/DGS10/downloaddata.

23. Oya Celasun and Geoffrey Keim, "The U.S. Federal Debt Outlook: Reading the Tea Leaves," Working Paper no. 10-62, International Monetary Fund, March 2010, http://core.kmi.open.ac.uk/download/pdf/6485598.pdf.

24. S. Ali Abbas, Nazim Belhocine, Asmaa A. ElGanainy, and Mark A. Hornton, "A Historical Public Debt Database," Working Paper no. 10-245, International Monetary Fund, November 2010.

25. Douglas Elmendorf and N. Gregory Mankiw, "Government Debt," Working Paper no. 6470, National Bureau of Economic Research, March 1998, pp. 18–21, http://www.nber.org/papers/w6470.pdf.

26. Ibid.

27. Theoretically, debt could be rolled over in perpetuity rather than being paid off. But that has the same effect as paying it off in present-value terms.

28. Elmendorf and Mankiw, "Government Debt," p. 20.

29. Roger C. Altman and Richard N. Haass, "American Profligacy and American Power: The Consequences of Fiscal Irresponsibility," *Foreign Affairs*, November–December 2010, http://www.foreignaffairs.com/articles/66778/roger-c-altman-and-richard-n-haass/american-profligacy-and-american-power.

30. Ibid.

31. Congressional Budget Office, "Federal Debt and the Risk of a Fiscal Crisis," Economic and Budget Issue Brief, July 2010, http://www.cbo.gov/sites/default/files/07-27_debt_fiscalcrisis_brief.pdf.

32. Zhou Xin, Simon Rabinovich, and Kevin Yao, "US Fiscal Health Worse than Europe: China Adviser," Reuters, December 8, 2010, http://www.reuters.com/article/2010/12/08/us-china-economy-growth-idUSTRE6B71KO20101208.

33. Elmendorf and Mankiw, "Government Debt," p. 21.

34. Federal Reserve Board, Department of the Treasury, "Major Foreign Holders of Treasury Securities," April 2014, http://www.treasury.gov/ticdata/Publish/mfh.txt.

35. Altman and Haass, "American Profligacy and American Power."

36. Charles T. Carlstrom and Jagadeesh Gokhale, "Government Consumption, Taxation, and Economic Activity," Federal Reserve Bank of Cleveland, 1991, p. 22, http://www.clevelandfed.org/research/review/1991/91-q3-carlstrom.pdf.

37. Congressional Budget Office, "The 2014 Long-Term Budget Outlook."

38. Congressional Budget Office, "The Budget and Economic Outlook: An Update," August 18, 2010, http://www.cbo.gov/sites/default/files/cbofiles/ftpdocs/117xx/doc11705/08-18-update.pdf; Amy Belasco, "The Cost of Iraq, Afghanistan, and Other Global War on Terror Operations Since 9/11," Congressional Research Service, RL33110, December 8, 2014, http://www.fas.org/sgp/crs/natsec/RL33110.pdf.

39. "How Much Did Bush Tax Cuts Cost in Forgone Revenue?" Tax Foundation, May 26, 2010, http://taxfoundation.org/article/how-much-did-bush-tax-cuts-cost -forgone-revenue. Note that figures for 2011 and 2012 have been extrapolated using their data.

40. Gregory Mankiw and Matthew Weinzierl, "Dynamic Scoring: A Back-of -the-Envelope Guide," Working Paper no. 11000, Harvard Institute of Economic Research, December 12, 2005, http://scholar.harvard.edu/files/mankiw/files /dynamicscoring_05-1212.pdf.

41. Congressional Budget Office, "Analyzing the Economic and Budgetary Effects of a 10 Percent Cut in Income Tax Rates," Economic and Budget Issue Brief, December 1, 2005.

42. "How Much Did Bush Tax Cuts Cost in Forgone Revenue?"; Congressional Budget Office, "The Budget and Economic Outlook: 2014 to 2024," February 2014, http://www.cbo.gov/sites/default/files/cbofiles/attachments/45010-Outlook2014 _Feb.pdf; Congressional Budget Office, "Historical Tables," September 17, 2013.

43. It has also been suggested that the current deficits are an unfortunate but necessary and temporary outgrowth of measures that are required to stimulate the economy in the face of a recession. That Keynesian approach holds that slow economic growth is caused by a decline in consumer demand, and that government should therefore stimulate consumer spending as a way to increase growth. As Paul Krugman and his coauthor Robin Wells argue, the key to economic recovery is for "the government to step in to spend when the private sector will not." Paul Krugman and Robin Wells, "The Way Out of the Slump," *New York Review of Books*, October 14, 2010. However, many economists question whether stimulating demand will actually boost economic growth. For example, University of Chicago economist Harald Uhlig calculates that stimulus spending similar to that of the American Recovery and Reinvestment Act results in $5.80 of output lost for each dollar spent on stimulus. Harald Uhlig, "Some Fiscal Calculus," *American Economic Review* 100, no. 2 (2010): 30–34. Even CBO director Douglas Elmendorf, who supported increased deficit spending as a stimulus measure, expressed concern that "fiscal policies that aim to increase demand are likely to decrease output and income in the long run because such policies usually increase government borrowing and reduce the nation's saving and capital stock." Douglas Elmendorf, director, Congressional Budget Office, "The Economic Outlook and Fiscal Policy Choices," Testimony before the Senate Committee on the Budget, 111th Cong., 2nd sess., September 28, 2010, p. 19, http://www.cbo.gov/sites/default/files /cbofiles/ftpdocs/118xx/doc11874/09-28-economicoutlook_testimony.pdf. Moreover, even if short-term deficit spending were beneficial, there is reason to be skeptical of Congress's ability to curtail such spending once the need has passed. As Elmendorf warned in his testimony, "If policies that widened the deficit in the near term were enacted, observers might question whether, when, and how the difficult actions to narrow the deficit later would be carried out" (p. 3).

44. James Gwartney, Robert Lawson, and Randall Holcombe, "The Size and Functions of Government and Economic Growth," Joint Economic Committee, April 1998, p. v, http://frihetspartiet.net/function.pdf.

45. Robert J. Barro, "Government Spending in a Simple Model of Endogenous Growth," *Journal of Political Economy* 98, no. 5 (1990): S122.

46. James S. Guseh, "Government Size and Economic Growth in Developing Countries: A Political-Economy Framework," *Journal of Macroeconomics* 19, no. 1 (January 1997): 175–92.

47. Stefan Fölster and Magnus Henrekson, "Growth Effects of Government Expenditure and Taxation in Rich Countries," Stockholm School of Economics, Working Paper Series in Economics and Finance, 2000.

48. Prmož Pevcin, "Does Optimal Size of Government Spending Exist?" University of Ljubljana, Slovenia, 2004, http://soc.kuleuven.be/io/egpa/fin/paper/slov2004/pevcin.pdf.

49. Gwartney, Lawson, and Holcombe, "Size and Functions of Government and Economic Growth." To be sure, not every study reaches the same conclusion. Perhaps the most widely cited of those contrary studies is a survey of 115 countries from 1960 to 1980 by Rati Ram of Illinois State University. Ram concluded that the impact of the size of government on economic output was almost always positive, though the relationship was possibly stronger in lower-income countries. Rati Ram, "Government Size and Economic Growth: A New Framework and Some Evidence from Cross-Section and Time Series Data," *American Economic Review* 76, no. 1 (1986): 191–203. However, as Eric Engen of the Federal Reserve Board and Jonathan Skinner of Dartmouth University point out in a paper for the National Bureau of Economic Research, "An obvious shortcoming with Ram's econometric estimates is endogeneity; countries that grow fast also tend to increase government spending." Eric M. Engen and Jonathan Skinner, "Fiscal Policy and Economic Growth," NBER Working paper no. 4223, National Bureau of Economic Research, December 1992, p. 7. That basically means that the direction of cause and effect cannot be properly determined from the selected variables, and it raises statistical problems with the concluding claim. In addition, both Jack Carr of the University of Texas and Bhaskara Rao of MIT criticize Ram's model for including government spending as part of GDP, which means that GDP may grow simply because government spending grows. Jack Carr, "Government Size and Economic Growth: A New Framework and Some Evidence from Cross-Section and Time Series Data, Comment," *American Economic Review* 76, no. 1 (1986): 267–71; Bhaskara Rao, "Government Size and Economic Growth: A New Framework and Some Evidence from Cross-Section and Time Series Data, Comment," *American Economic Review* 76, no. 1 (1986): 272–80.

50. Some might argue that the estimates of future GDP used to make the calculations in Figure 1.7 are too low, in part because the spending that the Obama administration is doing today is a form of "investment" that will lead to higher economic growth in the future. If GDP in the future is higher, then it follows that the ratio of spending to GDP will be lower than predicted. But although the evidence is not unambiguous, most studies suggest that, with the possible exception of spending on education and infrastructure, government expenditures add little to private productivity. See Paul Evans and Georgios Karras, "Are Government Activities Productive? Evidence from a Panel of U.S. States," *Review of Economics and Statistics* 76, no. 1 (February 1994): 1–11; Douglas Holtz-Eakin, "Public Sector Capital and the Productivity Puzzle," *Review of Economics and Statistics* 76, no. 1 (February 1994): 12–21; and Kevin Lansing, "Is Public Capital Productive? A Review of the Evidence," Federal Reserve Bank of Cleveland Economic Commentary, March 1, 1995. Moreover, as Figure 1.7 makes clear, the overwhelming majority of future spending increases monies from entitlement programs and interest on the debt, spending that is almost all consumption rather than investment. In addition, some might point out that a substantial portion of the projected future spending in Figure 1.7 is interest on the federal debt. Theoretically, if taxes were increased enough to cover spending, there would be no additional debt and therefore far lower interest payments. But even if one assumed

that the government accumulated no additional debt beyond the $13.4 trillion it currently owes, federal government spending would still exceed 30 percent of GDP by 2050. Throw in spending by state and local governments, and government spending would still consume half of the U.S. economy.

51. Carlstrom and Gokhale, "Government Consumption, Taxation, and Economic Activity."

52. Laffer himself warns: "The Laffer Curve itself does not say whether a tax cut will raise or lower revenues. Revenue responses to a tax rate change will depend upon the tax system in place, the time period being considered, the ease of movement into underground activities, the level of tax rates already in place, the prevalence of legal and accounting-driven tax loopholes, and the proclivities of the productive factors." Arthur Laffer, "The Laffer Curve: Past, Present, and Future," Backgrounder no. 1765, Heritage Foundation, June 1, 2004, p. 3, http://news.heartland.org/sites/all /modules/custom/heartland_migration/files/pdfs/15245. pdf.

53. Ibid.

54. Based on author's calculations using U.S. Census Bureau, "Statistical Abstract of the United States: 2012, Income Expenditures, Poverty, and Wealth," Table 717; Internal Revenue Service, SOI Tax Stats, Individual Income Tax Returns Filed and Sources of Income, "All Returns: Selected Income and Tax Items," Tax Year 2010, Table 1.1, http://www.irs.gov/uac/SOI-Tax-Stats---Individual-Statistical-Tables-by -Size-of-Adjusted-Gross-Income.

55. Letter from Peter R. Orszag, director, Congressional Budget Office, to the Honorable Paul Ryan, May 19, 2008, http://www.cbo.gov/sites/default/files/cbofiles /ftpdocs/92xx/doc9216/05-19-longtermbudget_letter-to-ryan.pdf.

56. Office of Management and Budget, "Guidelines and Discount Rates for Benefit–Cost Analysis of Federal Programs," Circular no. A-94 Revised, Transmittal Memo no. 64, October 29, 1992.

57. Congressional Budget Office, "Budget Options," February 2001, p. 381.

58. Martin Feldstein, "How Big Should Government Be?" *National Tax Journal* 50, no. 2 (June 1997): 211, http://ntj.tax.org/wwtax/ntjrec.nsf/notesview/36CFE3E5BC CB188C85256863004A5939/$file/v50n2197.pdf.

59. Congressional Budget Office, "Historical Budget Data: April 2014," April 14, 2014,Table 4, http://www.cbo.gov/sites/default/files/cbofiles/attachments/45249 -2014-04-HistoricalBudgetData.xlsx.

60. Congressional Budget Office, "Budget and Economic Outlook: 2014 to 2024."

61. Congressional Budget Office, "Historical Budget Data: April 2014."

62. Congressional Budget Office, "Budget and Economic Outlook: 2014 to 2024."

63. Congressional Budget Office, "The 2014 Long-Term Budget Outlook."

64. National Commission on Fiscal Responsibility and Reform, "The Moment of Truth."

65. Ed Hornick, "Democrats to Use Social Security against GOP This Fall," CNN.com, August 13, 2010, http://www.cnn.com/2010/POLITICS/08/13 /democrats.social.security/.

66. Angie Drobnic Holan, "Politifact: Republican Exaggerations about Cutting Medicare," *Tampa Bay Times*, October 11, 2010, http://www.politifact.com/truth-o-meter /article/2010/oct/11/republican-exaggerations-about-cutting-medicare.

Chapter 2

1. European Commission, "General Government Gross Debt," Eurostat Database, http://epp.eurostat.ec.europa.eu/tgm/refreshTableAction.do?tab=table&plugin=l& pcode=teina230&language=en.

2. European Commission "General Government Deficit/Surplus," Eurostat Database, http://epp.eurostat.ec.europa.eu/tgm/table.do?tab=table&init=l&language =en&pcode=tec00127&plugin=l.

3. European Commission, "General Government Gross Debt"; Organisation for Economic Co-operation and Development, "Public Sector Debt: Consolidated, Nominal Value," http://stats.oecd.org/index.aspx?queryid=350.

4. European Commission, "General Government Gross Debt"; European Commission, "Enlargement: Croatia," http://ec.europa.eu/enlargement/countries/detailed -country-information/croatia/index_en.

5. Ibid.

6. S. Ali Abbas, Nazim Belhocine, Asmaa ElGanainy, and Mark Horton, "A Historical Public Debt Database," Working Paper no. 10-245, International Monetary Fund, November 2010, https://www.imf.org/external/pubs/cat/longres.cfm?sk=24332.0.

7. Sarah Levy, "Pensions in the National Accounts: A Fuller Picture of the UK's Funded and Unfunded Pension Obligations," UK Office for National Statistics, Pensions Analysis Unit, April 27, 2012, http://www.ons.gov.uk/ons/rel/pensions /pensions-in-the-national-accounts/uk-national-accounts-supplementary-table-on -pensions--2010-/art-mainarticle.html.

8. Jagadeesh Gokhale, "Measuring the Unfunded Liabilities of European Countries," Policy Report no. 319, National Center for Policy Analysis, January 2009, http://www.ncpa.org/pdfs/st319.pdf.

9. Jagadeesh Gokhale and Erin Partin, "Europe and the United States: On the Fiscal Brink?" *Cato Journal* 33, no. 2 (Spring–Summer 2013): 193–210, http://object.cato.org /sites/cato.org/files/serials/files/cato-journal/2013/5/cj33n2-1.pdf.

10. Author's calculations using European Commission, "General Government Gross Debt"; European Commission, "Population on 1 January," Eurostat Database; Treasury Direct, "Debt to the Penny and Who Holds It," http://www.treasurydirect .gov/NP/debt/current.

11. International Monetary Fund, "Currency Composition of Official Foreign Exchange Reserves (GOFER)," 2013, https://www.imf.org/external/np/sta/cofer /eng/index.htm.

12. Craig K. Elwell, "The Depreciating Dollar: Economic Effects and Policy Response," Congressional Research Service, February 23, 2012, p. 6.

13. Congressional Budget Office, "Federal Debt and the Risk of a Fiscal Crisis," Economic and Budget Issue Brief, July 27, 2010, p. 1, http://www.cbo.gov/sites /default/files/cbofiles/ftpdocs/116xx/doc11659/07-27_debt_fiscalcrisis_brief.pdf.

14. Author's calculations using information from Federal Reserve Bank of St. Louis, "H.15 Selected Interest Rates: 10-Year Treasury Constant Maturity Rate (DGS10)," http://research.stlouisfed.org/fred2/series/DGS10/downloaddata.

15. Doug Elmendorf, "How Different Future Interest Rates Would Affect Budget Deficits," Congressional Budget Office, March 27, 2013, Table 2, http://www.cbo. gov/publication/44024.

16. Marvin Goodfriend, "Interest Rate Policy and the Inflation Scare Problem 1979–1992," Federal Reserve Bank of Richmond, *Economic Quarterly* 79, no. 1 (Winter 1993): 1–23.

17. Congressional Budget Office, "Federal Debt and the Risk of a Fiscal Crisis," p. 7.

18. Standard & Poor's Ratings Services, "Sovereign Ratings List," http://www .standardandpoors.com/ratings/sovereigns/ratings-list/en/us?sectorName =null&subSectorCode=.

19. Government Accountability Office, "State and Local Governments' Fiscal Outlook: April 2012 Update," April 5, 2012, http://www.gao.gov/assets/590/589908 .pdf; Congressional Budget Office, "Long-Term Budget Outlook 2013: Supplementary Tables," September 17, 2013, http://www.cbo.gov/sites/default/files/cbofiles /attachments/45308-2013-09-LTBOSuppData.xlsx; European Commission, "Government Expenditure, Revenue and Main Aggregates," Eurostat Database, http:// appsso.eurostat.ec.europa.eu/nui/show.do?dataset=gov_a_main&lang=en.

Chapter 3

1. Paul Krugman, "The Mostly Solved Deficit Problem," *New York Times*, January 10, 2013, http://krugman.blogs.nytimes.com/2013/01/10/the-mostly-solved-deficit -problem/?_php=true&_type=blogs&_r=0.

2. Matt Yglesias, "There Is No Sovereign Debt Crisis," *Slate*, July 25, 2012, http:// www.slate.com/articles/business/moneybox/2012/07/there_is_no_sovereign_debt _crisis_most_governments_have_never_been_able_to_borrow_so_cheaply.html.

3. Bruce Bartlett, "Why Government Spending Is Not Out of Control," *Fiscal Times*, January 25, 2013, http://www.thefiscaltimes.com/Columns/2013/01/25 /Why-Government-Spending-Is-Not-Out-of-Control.

4. John Maynard Keynes, *The Collected Writings: Activities, 1922–29—The Return to Gold and Industrial Policy, Part II*, vol. 19 (collected works of Keynes), ed. D. E. Moggridge (London: Macmillan, 1981).

5. Paul Krugman, "Debt Is (Mostly) Money We Owe to Ourselves," *New York Times*, December 28, 2011, http://krugman.blogs.nytimes.com/2011/12/28/debt-is -mostly-money-we-owe-to-ourselves.

6. James M. Buchanan, *The Collected Works of James M. Buchanan*, vol. 2, *Public Principles of Public Debt: A Defense and Restatement* (Indianapolis: Liberty Fund, 1999), http://oll.libertyfund.org/title/279/31085.

7. Of course, even advocates of "we owe it to ourselves" make a distinction between domestic and foreign-held debt. And, as noted in Chapter 1, roughly 48 percent of our current national debt is held by foreign countries and institutions, though Krugman notes that the United States has offsetting claims against foreigners, roughly 89 cents in claims for every dollar we owe. Even so, that is not quite the same thing.

8. Buchanan, *Collected Works*.

9. Ludwig von Mises, *Human Action* (Indianapolis: Liberty Fund, 1996).

10. Buchanan, *Collected Works*.

11. Ibid. (emphasis in original).

12. Congressional Budget Office, "Federal Investment," December 18, 2013, http:// www.cbo.gov/sites/default/files/cbofiles/attachments/44974-FederalInvestment.pdf.

13. Author's calculations based on data from Congressional Budget Office, "The Budget and Economic Outlook: 2014 to 2024," February 2014, Table 3.1, http://www.cbo.gov/sites/default/files/cbofiles/attachments/45010-Outlook2014_Feb.pdf.

14. Arnold Kling, "Lenders and Spenders: Confronting the Political Reality of Debt," *The American*, November 20, 2012, http://www.american.com/archive/2012/november/lenders-and-spenders-confronting-the-political-reality-of-debt.

15. Peter R. Orszag and William G. Gale, "Budget Deficits, National Saving, and Interest Rates," Brookings Institution, September 2004, http://www.brookings.edu/research/papers/2004/09/budgetdeficit-gale.

16. Buchanan, *Collected Works*.

17. Bureau of Economic Analysis, "National Income and Product Accounts Tables," Table 1.1.1, http://www.bea.gov/national/txt/dpga.txt.

18. Bureau of Labor Statistics, "Household Data," Table A-1, http://www.bls.gov/news.release/empsit.t01.htm.

19. John Maynard Keynes, *The General Theory of Employment, Interest and Money* (London: Palgrave Macmillan, 1936), chap. 13, 15, and 17, http://cas.umkc.edu/economics/people/facultypages/kregel/courses/econ645/winter2011/generaltheory.pdf.

20. Henry Farrell and John Quiggin, "How to Save the Euro—and the EU: Reading Keynes in Brussels," *Foreign Affairs*, May–June 2011, http://www.foreignaffairs.com/articles/67761/henry-farrell-and-john-quiggin/how-to-save-the-euro-and-the-eu.

21. Huberto M. Ennis and Alexander L. Wolman, "Large Excess Reserves in the U.S.: A View from the Cross-Section of Banks," Working Paper no. 12-05, Federal Reserve Bank of Richmond, August 2012, https://www.richmondfed.org/publications/research/working_papers/2012/pdf/wp12-05.pdf.

22. Robert Pollin, "The Great U.S. Liquidity Trap of 2009–11: Are We Stuck Pushing on Strings?" Political Economy Research Institute, University of Massachusetts Amherst, June 2012, p. 2, http://www.peri.umass.edu/fileadmin/pdf/working_papers/working_papers_251-300/WP284.pdf.

23. Paul Krugman, "The Stimulus Tragedy," *New York Times*, February 21, 2014, http://www.nytimes.com/2014/02/21/opinion/krugman-the-stimulus-tragedy.html?_r=0.

24. The Federal Reserve Bank of Minneapolis, "The Recession and Recovery in Perspective," http://www.minneapolisfed.org/publications/special-studies/rip/recession-in-perspective.

25. Ibid.

26. Robert Samuelson, "Economists in the Dark," *Washington Post*, February 16, 2014, http://www.washingtonpost.com/opinions/robert-samuelson-economists-face-hard-times/2014/02/16/70991824-9599-11e3-afce-3e7c922ef31e_story.html.

27. Paul Krugman, interview on *Fareed Zakaria GPS*, CNN, August 12, 2011, http://globalpublicsquare.blogs.cnn.com/2011/08/12/gps-this-sunday-krugman-calls-for-space-aliens-to-fix-u-s-economy.

28. Bill Dupor, "The 2009 Recovery Act: Directly Created and Saved Jobs Were Primarily in Government," Federal Reserve Bank of St. Louis, *Review* 96, no. 2 (2014): 123, http://research.stlouisfed.org/publications/review/2014/q2/dupor.pdf.

29. Christopher Flavelle and Jeff Larson, "Stimulus: How Fast We're Spending Nearly $800 Billion," ProPublica, http://projects.propublica.org/tables/stimulus-spending-progress.

30. Alan Chernoff, "Where's the Stimulus?" CNN, February 17, 2011, http://money.cnn.com/2011/02/17/news/economy/stimulus_bill.

31. Robert J. Barro, "Are Government Bonds Net Wealth?" *Journal of Political Economy* 82, no. 6 (November–December 1974): 1095–117.

32. David Ricardo, "Essay on the Funding System," in *The Works of David Ricardo: With a Notice of the Life and Writings of the Author*, collected by J. R. McCulloch (London: John Murray, 1888).

33. Juan M. Sanchez and Emrican Yurdagul, "Why Are Corporations Holding So Much Cash?" Federal Reserve Bank of St. Louis, January 2013, https://www.stlouisfed.org/Publications/Regional-Economist/January-2013/Why-Are-Corporations-Holding-So-Much-Cash.

34. Alessandro Turrini, "Fiscal Policy and the Cycle in the Euro Area: The Role of Government Revenue and Expenditure," European Commission, Economic Papers 323, April 2008, http://ec.europa.eu/economy_finance/publications/publication12600_en.pdf.

35. Lawrence Summers, "Breaking the Negative Feedback Loop," *Reuters*, June 3, 2012, http://blogs.reuters.com/lawrencesummers/2012/06/03/breaking-the-negative-feedback-loop.

36. Matt Yglesias, "Borrow. Borrow. And Borrow Some More," *Slate*, December 5, 2011, http://www.slate.com/articles/business/moneybox/2011/12/raise_taxes_cut_spending_borrow_more_one_of_these_fiscal_strategies_is_clearly_best_which_one_.html.

37. Congressional Budget Office, "Updated Budget Projections: 2014 to 2024," April 2014, http://www.cbo.gov/sites/default/files/cbofiles/attachments/45229-UpdatedBudgetProjections_2.pdf.

38. Committee for a Responsible Federal Budget, "Understanding the Sequester," November 13, 2013; Congressional Budget Office, "Budget and Economic Outlook: 2014 to 2024." The Continuing Resolution for 2014 spending levels set spending above the caps put in place by the sequester, reversing some of the cuts that would have taken effect.

39. Jonathan Spicer and Jason Lange, "Yellen Stays the Course, says Fed to Keep Trimming Stimulus," *Reuters*, February 11, 2014, http://www.reuters.com/article/2014/02/11/us-usa-fed-idUSBREA1A06O20140211.

40. U.S. Department of the Treasury, "Daily Treasury Yield Curve Rates," January 9, 2015, http://www.treasury.gov/resource-center/data-chart-center/interest-rates/Pages/TextView.aspx?data=yield.

41. Congressional Budget Office, "CBO's Projections of Federal Interest Payments," September 3, 2014.

42. Congressional Budget Office, "The 2014 Long-Term Budget Outlook," August 27, 2014; Congressional Budget Office, "An Update to the Budget and Economic Outlook: 2014 to 2024," August 27, 2024.

43. Congressional Budget Office, "An Update to the Budget and Economic Outlook: 2014 to 2024."

44. Ibid.

45. Congressional Budget Office, "Updated Budget Projections: Fiscal Years 2013 to 2023," May 2013 http://www.cbo.gov/sites/default/files/44172-Baseline2.pdf; Congressional Budget Office, "An Update to the Budget and Economic Outlook: 2014 to 2024."

46. House Budget Committee, "Summary of the Bipartisan Budget Act of 2013," December 10, 2013, http://budget.house.gov/uploadedfiles/bba2013summary.pdf.

47. Author's calculations based on estimates in letter from Peter R. Orszag, director, Congressional Budget Office, to the Honorable Tom Harkin on H.R. 2419, the Food, Conservation, and Energy Act of 2008, May 13, 2008; and letter from Douglas W. Elmendorf, director, Congressional Budget Office, to the Honorable Frank D. Lucas on H.R. 2642, Agricultural Act of 2014, January 28, 2014, http://www.cbo .gov/sites/default/files/cbofiles/attachments/hr2642LucasLtr.pdf.

48. Author's calculations based on estimates in Office of Management and Budget, "Fiscal Year 2015 Budget of the U.S. Government," March 4, 2014, http://www .whitehouse.gov/sites/default/files/omb/budget/fy2015/assets/budget.pdf; and Congressional Budget Office, "Budget and Economic Outlook: 2014 to 2024."

49. Ibid.

50. Office of Management and Budget, "Fiscal Year 2015 Budget," p. 30.

51. Author's calculations using Office of Management and Budget, "Fiscal Year 2015 Budget," March 4, 2014, Table S-13.

52. Matt Yglesias, "In the Long Run . . .," *Slate*, March 20, 2012, http://www.slate .com/blogs/moneybox/2012/03/20/in_the_long_run_.html.

53. Stephen Dinan, "Entitlements Have History of Cost Overruns," *Washington Times*, June 25, 2003, http://www.washingtontimes.com/news/2003/jun /25/20030625-115757-6676r/?page=all.

54. Ibid.

55. Ibid. In fairness, it should be pointed out that, so far, Medicare Part D is costing less than estimated.

56. Greenspan Commission, "Report of the National Commission on Social Security Reform," January 1983, http://www.ssa.gov/history/reports/gspan.html.

57. *The 2014 Annual Report of the Board of Trustees of the Federal Old-Age and Survivors Insurance and Federal Disability Insurance Trust Funds* (Washington: Government Printing Office, July 28, 2014), http ://www. ssa.gov/oact/tr/2014/tr2014.pdf.

58. Congressional Budget Office, "Budget and Economic Outlook: 2014 to 2024"; Congressional Budget Office, "The Budget and Economic Outlook: Fiscal Years 2013 to 2023," February 2013; letter from Douglas W. Elmendorf, director, Congressional Budget Office, to the Honorable Nancy Pelosi on H.R. 4872, The Reconciliation Act, March 20, 2010, http://www.cbo.gov/publication/45231.

Chapter 4

1. NBC News, "Full Video and Transcript of Leaked Romney Fundraiser Remarks," September 19, 2012, http://firstread.nbcnews.com/_news/2012/09/18/13943563 -full-video-and-transcript-of-leaked-romney-fundraiser-remarks?lite.

2. Tax Policy Center, "T13-0231- Distribution of Tax Units That Pay No Individual Income Tax: By Expanded Cash Income Level, Current Law, 2014," August 29, 2013.

3. Will Freeland, William McBride, and Ed Gerrish, "The Fiscal Costs of Nonpayers," Special Report no. 203, Tax Foundation, September 19, 2012, http://taxfoundation.org /article/fiscal-costs-nonpayers.

4. Ibid.

5. Alec MacGillis, "Obama's '70 Million Checks' per Month: Actually, It's Even More than That," *Washington Post*, July 26, 2011, http://www.washingtonpost.com/politics

/obamas-70-million-checks-per-month-actually-its-even-more-than-that/2011/07/26
/gIQAT3XkbI_story.html.

6. Congressional Budget Office, "The Distribution of Household Income and Federal Taxes, 2011," November 12, 2014.

7. Scott A. Hodge and Gerald Prante, "The Distribution of Tax and Spending Policies in the United States," Tax Foundation, Special Report No. 211, November 18, 2013, http://taxfoundation.org/article/distribution-tax-and-spending-policies-united-states.

8. Bureau of Economic Analysis, "National Income and Product Accounts Tables," Table 2.1.

9. Daniel Indiviglio, "Is the U.S. Becoming a Welfare State?" *Atlantic*, March 9, 2011, http://www.theatlantic.com/business/archive/2011/03/is-the-us-becoming-a-welfare-state/72217/.

10. Author's calculations using Bureau of Economic Analysis, "National Income and Product Accounts Tables," Table 2.1; Office of Management and Budget, "Historical Tables," Table 1.1, http://www.whitehouse.gov/omb/budget/historicals; and Federal Reserve Bank of St. Louis, Economic Data, "State and Local Government Total Expenditures" (W079RC1A027NBEA), https://research.stlouisfed.org/fred2/series/W079RC1A027NBEA/downloaddata.

11. Congressional Budget Office, "The Distribution of Household Income and Federal Taxes, 2011," Sources of Income for All Households, by Market Income Group, 1979 to 2011,Table 7.

12. Congressional Budget Office, "An Update to the Budget and Economic Outlook: 2014 to 2024," August 27, 2014.

13. Ibid.

14. Office of Management and Budget, "Historical Tables," Table 8.4, http://www.whitehouse.gov/omb/budget/historicals.

15. International Monetary Fund, "5. Report for Selected Countries," World Economic Outlook Database, April 2013.

16. Congressional Budget Office, "2014 Long-Term Budget Outlook," July 25, 2014, http://www.cbo.gov/sites/default/files/cbofiles/attachments/45308-2014-07-LTBOSuppData_update2.xlsx. (Note that Medicaid spending also includes ACA subsidies through the Exchanges. The CBO does not list subsidy spending separately.)

17. Congressional Budget Office, "Effects of the Affordable Care Act on Health Insurance Coverage: Baseline Projections," April 14, 2014; Congressional Budget Office, "Updated Budget Projections: 2014 to 2024," April 2014, http://www.cbo.gov/sites/default/files/cbofiles/attachments/45229-UpdatedBudgetProjections_2.pdf.

18. Bipartisan Commission on Entitlement and Tax Reform, 1995, *Final Report to the President* (Washington: Government Printing Office/Diane Publishing, 1995).

19. National Bipartisan Commission on the Future of Medicare, "Building a Better Medicare for Today and Tomorrow," March 1999.

20. "Report of the 1994–1996 Advisory Council on Social Security," vol. 1, "Findings and Recommendations," Social Security Administration, January 1997, http://www.ssa.gov/history/reports/adcouncil/report/toc.htm.

21. Ed Hornick, "Democrats to Use Social Security against GOP This Fall," CNN .com, August 13, 2010, http://www.cnn.com/2010/POLITICS/08/13/democrats .social.security.

22. Angie Drobnic Holan, "Politifact: Republican Exaggerations about Cutting Medicare," *Tampa Bay Times*, October 11, 2010, http://www.politifact.com/truth -o-meter/article/2010/oct/11/republican-exaggerations-about-cutting-medicare.

23. Nicholas Eberstadt, *A Nation of Takers: America's Entitlement Epidemic* (West Conshohocken, PA: Templeton Press, 2012), p. 23.

24. Social Security Administration, "Income of the Population 55 or Older, 2012," March 2012, Table 2.A1, http://www.ssa.gov/policy/docs/statcomps/income_pop55 /2012/sect02.html#table2.a1.

25. Centers for Medicare and Medicaid Services, "Seniors and Medicare and Medic- aid Enrollees," Department of Health and Human Services, http://www.medicaid.gov /Medicaid-CHIP-Program-Information/By-Population/Medicare-Medicaid-Enrollees -Dual-Eligibles/Seniors-and-Medicare-and-Medicaid-Enrollees.html.

26. Social Security Administration, "Income of the Population 55 or Older, 2012."

27. Ibid.

28. Centers for Medicare and Medicaid Services, "National Health Expendi- ture Data: Age and Gender Tables," Department of Health and Human Services, http://www.cms.gov/Research-Statistics-Data-and-Systems/Statistics-Trends-and -Reports/NationalHealthExpendData/Downloads/2010GenderandAgeTables.pdf.

29. Ibid.

30. Kaiser Family Foundation, "Medicaid's Role in Meeting the Long-Term Care Needs of American Seniors," Kaiser Commission on Medicaid and the Uninsured, January 2013, http://kaiserfamilyfoundation.files.wordpress.com/2013/02/8403.pdf.

31. U.S. Census Bureau, "Voting and Registration in the Election of November 2012—Detailed Tables," November 2012, Table 1, http://www.census.gov/hhes /www/socdemo/voting//publications/p20/2012/Table01.xls.

Chapter 5

1. Rick Perry, *Fed Up: Our Fight to Save America from Washington* (New York: Little, Brown, 2010), p. 171.

2. Ibid., p. 61.

3. There is much debate over the question of whether "return" is an accurate con- cept when discussing Social Security benefits received versus taxes paid. We don't, for example, consider whether defense spending provides a "return" on income taxes paid. And despite the implication—frequently abetted by politicians—that Social Security benefits are in some way related to Social Security taxes, the Supreme Court has twice ruled that they are not. *Flemming v. Nestor*, 363 U.S. 603 (1960); *Helvering v. Davis*, 301 U.S. 619 (1937). Other experts, such as former Social Security administrator Robert J. Myers, author of the preeminent textbook on Social Security, suggest that "rate of return accurately applies to the portion of the payroll tax paid by the indi- vidual worker, but not to the portion paid by the employer." Robert J. Myers, *Social Security*, 3rd ed. (Burr Ridge, IL: Irwin, 1985). However, many other experts from across the political spectrum, including this author, continue to view the term as the best measure of benefits versus contributions and a way to make such comparisons with private investments.

4. Milton Friedman, "The Biggest Ponzi Scheme on Earth," *Hoover Digest*, no. 2 (April 1999), http://www.hoover.org/research/biggest-ponzi-scheme-earth.

5. Paul Samuelson, "Social Security Is a Ponzi Scheme That Works," *Newsweek*, February 13, 1967, cited by Alex Tabarrok in "Is Social Security a Ponzi Scheme?" Marginal Revolution (blog), September 10, 2011, http://marginalrevolution.com /marginalrevolution/2011/09/is-social-security-a-ponzi-scheme.html.

6. Paul R. Krugman, "What Consensus?" *Boston Review*, December–January 1996–97, http://new.bostonreview.net/BR21.6/krugmann.html.

7. Social Security Administration, "Contribution and Benefit Base," http://www.ssa .gov/oact/COLA/cbb.html#Series.

8. "Carter Signs Social Security Tax Rise for 110 Million," *New York Times*, December 21, 1977, p. A19.

9. Greenspan Commission, "Report of the National Commission on Social Security Reform," January 1983, http://www.ssa.gov/history/reports/gspan.html.

10. Office of Management and Budget, "Fiscal Year 2014 Budget of the U.S. Government," 2013, p. 46, http://www.gpo.gov/fdsys/pkg/BUDGET-2014-BUD/pdf /BUDGET-2014-BUD.pdf.

11. Michael D. Shear, "Obama's Budget Omits Trims to Social Security," *New York Times*, February 20, 2014, http://www.nytimes.com/2014/02/21/us/politics /obamas-2015- budget-to-sidestep-bipartisan-offers.html?_r=0.

12. *The 2014 Annual Report of the Board of Trustees of the Federal Old-Age and Survivors Insurance and Federal Disability Insurance Trust Funds* (Washington: Government Printing Office, July 28, 2014), Tables III.A5, IV.B2, http://www.ssa.gov/oact/tr/2014 /tr2014.pdf.

13. Social Security Administration, "Income of the Population 55 or Older, 2010," Office of Research, Evaluation, and Statistics; Office of Retirement and Disability Policy, March, 2012, Table 10.1, http://www.ssa.gov/policy/docs/statcomps/income _pop55/2012/sect02.html#table2.a1.

14. Ibid.

15. Dawn Nuschler, "Social Security Primer," Congressional Research Service, June 17, 2013, https://www.fas.org/sgp/crs/misc/R42035.pdf.

16. Social Security Administration, "Benefit Formula Bend Points," 2014, http:// www.ssa.gov/oact/cola/bendpoints.html.

17. Social Security Administration, "Effect of Early or Delayed Retirement on Retirement Benefits," 2010, http://www.ssa.gov/oact/ProgData/ar_drc.html.

18. Nuschler, "Social Security Primer."

19. *2014 Annual Report*, Tables III.A5, IV.B2.

20. The monthly benefit cap formula is 150 percent of the first $980 of the PIA, plus 272 percent of the PIA between $980 and $1,415 per month, 134 percent of the PIA between $1,416 and $1,845, and 175 percent of the PIA above $1,845. Nuschler, "Social Security Primer."

21. *2014 Annual Report*.

22. Social Security Administration, "How Workers' Compensation and Other Disability Payments May Affect Your Benefits," SSA Publication no. 05-10018, January 2011, http://www.ssa.gov/pubs/EN-05-10018.pdf.

23. Thomas F. Siems, "Reengineering Social Security for the New Economy," Cato Institute Project on Social Security Privatization, SSP no. 22, January 23, 2001, http:// www.cato.org/sites/cato.org/files/pubs/pdf/ssp22.pdf.

24. *2014 Annual Report*.

25. Ibid., Table II.B.2.

26. That does not technically constitute a deficit because Social Security also received $105.7 billion in interest payments on the bonds in the trust fund and $30.9 billion in general revenue reimbursements as compensation for the temporary payroll tax reduction passed in 2010 and renewed in 2011. However, even considering those payments, Social Security will run a cash-flow deficit by 2020. *2014 Annual Report*, Table II.B.2.

27. Ibid., Table II.B.2. This is just the initial cut. The reductions rise over time, reaching 29 percent by 2087.

28. Ibid.

29. Executive Office of the President, *Budget of the United States Government, Fiscal Year 2000: Analytical Perspectives* (Washington: Government Printing Office, 1999), p. 337, http://www.gpo.gov/fdsys/pkg/BUDGET-2000-PER/pdf/BUDGET-2000-PER.pdf.

30. Discounted present value of Social Security's liabilities over an infinite horizon. *2014 Annual Report*, p. 6.

31. Ibid.

32. Social Security Administration, "Your Social Security Statement," http://www.ssa .gov/myaccount/materials/pdfs/SSA-7005-OL.pdf.

33. *Flemming v. Nestor*, 363 U.S. 603 (1960).

34. *Helvering v. Davis*, 301 U.S. 619 (1937).

35. William Jefferson Clinton, "Remarks by the President via Satellite to the Regional Congressional Social Security Forums," Albuquerque, NM, July 27, 1998, http://www.ssa.gov/history/clntstmts.html#forum72798.

36. Social Security Administration, "Contribution and Benefit Base," http://www.ssa.gov/oact/cola/cbb.html.

37. *The 1993 Annual Report of the Board of Trustees of the Federal Old-Age and Survivors Insurance and Federal Disability Insurance Trust Funds* (Washington: Government Printing Office, May 1993).

38. For Generation 0 (the currently retired population), nothing has been accumulated, so they must rely on private savings and pensions. Siems, "Reengineering Social Security."

39. In 2005, actuaries with the Social Security Administration scored a proposal by scholars from the Cato Institute that combines the wage–price indexing proposal described here with personal accounts equal to 6.2 percent of wages as reducing Social Security's unfunded liabilities by $6.3 trillion, roughly half the system's predicted shortfall at that time. If the Cato plan had been adopted in 2005, the system would have begun running surpluses by 2046. Indeed, by the end of the 75-year actuarial window, the system would have been running surpluses in excess of $1.8 trillion. Michael Tanner, "A Better Deal at Half the Cost: SSA Scoring of the Cato Plan for Social Security Reform," Cato Institute Briefing Paper no. 92, April 25, 2005. At the same time, SSA actuaries concluded that average-wage workers who were 45 or younger could expect higher benefits under the Cato proposal than Social Security would otherwise be able to pay. Although no more current scoring is available, there is no reason to presume that savings or benefits would be substantially different today.

40. Michael Tanner, "Still a Better Deal: Private Investment vs. Social Security," Cato Institute Policy Analysis no. 692, February 13, 2012, http://www.cato.org /sites/cato.org/files/pubs/pdf/PA692.pdf.

41. Ibid.

42. Ibid. It is worth restating that 2011 was near the low point of the stock market, almost a "worst-case scenario" for retirees. People retiring three years later than the study's cohort—so people retiring in 2014—would have enjoyed compound annual growth rate returns of 15.88 percent in 2012 and 32.42 percent in 2013, which was the highest one-year return since 1997. The point is that those people would have enjoyed even higher returns than the ones found in the Cato study.

43. Ibid.

44. C. Eugene Steurle, Karen E. Smith, and Caleb Quakenbush, "Has Social Security Redistributed to Whites from People of Color?" Program on Retirement Policy Brief no. 38, Urban Institute, November 2013, http://www.urban.org/UploadedPDF/412943 -Has-Social-Security-Redistributed-to-Whites-from-People-of-Color.pdf.

45. Thomas Piketty, *Capital in the Twenty-First Century*, trans. Arthur Goldhammer (Cambridge, MA: Belknap Press, 2014), p. 571.

46. José Piñera, "Toward a World of Worker-Capitalists," Cato Institute, April 11, 2001, http://www.cato.org/publications/commentary/toward-world-workercapitalists.

47. Jagadeesh Gokhale, "Social Security Reform, Does Privatization Still Make Sense?" *Harvard Law School Journal on Legislation* 50, no. 1 (2013): 169–207.

48. Martin Feldstein, "Privatizing Social Security: The $10 Trillion Opportunity," Cato Institute Project on Social Security Privatization, SSP no. 7, January 31, 1997, http://www.cato.org/pubs/ssps/ssp7.html.

49. See, for example, the "scoring" of Cato's proposal for personal accounts. Tanner, "A Better Deal at Half the Cost."

Chapter 6

1. Congressional Budget Office, "Medicare, April 2014 Baseline," April 14, 2014. The August update does not have a Medicare baseline that breaks down Medicare projections into different components. As such, we continue to use the April baseline.

2. David Dranove, Craig Garthwaite, and Christopher Ody, "Health Spending Slowdown Is Mostly Due to Economic Factors, Not Structural Change in the Health Care Sector," *Health Affairs* 33, no. 8 (2014): 1399–1406.

3. Kaiser Family Foundation, "Assessing the Effects of the Economy on the Recent Slowdown in Health Spending," April 22, 2013, http://kff.org/health-costs/issue -brief/assessing-the-effects-of-the-economy-on-the-recent-slowdown-in-health -spending-2/. It should be noted that another study by David Cutler and Nikhil Sahni in Health Affairs found that the recession explained only 37 percent of the slowdown, but 55 percent of the slowdown remained unexplained. David M. Cutler and Nikhil R. Sahni, "If Slow Rate of Health Care Spending Growth Persists, Projections May Be Off by $770 Billion," *Health Affairs* 32, no. 5 (2013): 841–50.

4. Congressional Budget Office, "April 2014 Medicare Baseline by Fiscal Year," April 14, 2014, http://www.cbo.gov/sites/default/files/cbofiles/attachments/44205-2014 -04-Medicare.pdf.

5. Letter from Douglas W. Elmendorf, director, Congressional Budget Office, to the Honorable Nancy Pelosi on H.R. 4872, the Reconciliation Act of 2010, March 20, 2010, https://www.cbo.gov/sites/default/files/cbofiles/ftpdocs/113xx/doc11379 /amendreconprop.pdf.

6. Centers for Medicare and Medicaid Services, "National Health Expenditure Data for 1960–2013," Table 1, http://www.cms.gov/Research-Statistics-Data-and-Systems /Statistics-Trends-and-Reports/NationalHealthExpendData/downloads/tables.pdf.

7. Congressional Budget Office, "April 2014 Medicare Baseline."

8. That is assuming an individual's income is less than $85,000, or joint filers have income of less than $170,000. Premiums are adjusted for income level; higher incomes would face higher premiums, up to $335.70 for individuals with more than $214,000 and joint filers with more than $428,000.

9. Congressional Budget Office, "April 2014 Medicare Baseline."

10. Ibid.

11. *2014 Annual Report of the Boards of Trustees of the Federal Hospital Insurance and Federal Supplementary Medical Insurance Trust Funds* (Baltimore: Centers for Medicare and Medicaid Services, July 28, 2014), Table III.D3, http://www.cms.gov/Research -Statistics-Data-and-Systems/Statistics-Trends-and-Reports/ReportsTrustFunds /downloads/tr2014.pdf.

12. Kaiser Family Foundation, "The Medicare Part D Prescription Drug Benefit," fact sheet, November 2013, http://kaiserfamilyfoundation.files.wordpress .com/2013/11/7044-14-medicare-part-d-fact-sheet.pdf.

13. Elmendorf, letter to the Honorable Nancy Pelosi on H.R. 4872.

14. However, drug companies expect to more than make up this cost from other provisions in the bill, such as expanded insurance coverage and an inclusion of prescription drugs, in the minimal acceptable coverage mandate. As a result, the pharmaceutical industry strongly supported the bill's passage.

15. The author is not opposed to all third-party payment. The idea of a third party helping spread risk is fundamental to the concept of insurance. However, it cannot be denied that third-party payment distorts use patterns and increases costs. See Robert H. Brook et al., "The Health Insurance Experiment: A Classic RAND Study Speaks to the Current Health Care Reform Debate," RAND Corporation, 2006, http://www.rand.org/pubs/research_briefs/RB9174.html; and Stan Liebowitz, "Why Health Care Costs Too Much," Cato Institute Policy Analysis no. 211, June 23, 1994, http://www.cato.org/pubs/pas/pa211.html. That is not to say that there should be no insurance (or third-party payment), but an overreliance on third-party payment, especially for routine care, has consequences with regard to cost. That result is exacerbated when third-party payment is subsidized, as in Medicare.

16. U.S. Census Bureau, "2012 Statistical Abstract of the United States," Table 104.

17. U.S. Census Bureau, "2012 National Population Projections," Tables 3, 12.

18. Ibid.

19. Congressional Budget Office, "April 2014 Medicare Baseline."

20. U.S. Department of Health and Human Services, "The High Concentration of U.S. Health Care Expenditures," Research in Action Issue no. 19, Agency for Healthcare and Research Quality.

21. Lauren Wier, Anne Pfuntner, and Claudia Steiner, "Hospital Utilization among Oldest Adults, 2008," Statistical Brief no. 103, Healthcare Cost and Utilization Project, Agency for Healthcare Research and Quality; Donald Cherry, Christine Lucas, and Sandra L. Decker, "Population Aging and the Use of Office-Based Physician Services," NCHS Data Brief no. 41, August 2010, National Center for Health Statistics, U.S. Department of Health and Human Services.

22. Ibid.

23. Berhanu Alemayehu and Kenneth E. Warner, "The Lifetime Distribution of Health Care Costs," *Health Services Research* 39, no. 3 (2004): 627–42.

24. Congressional Budget Office, "Technological Change and the Growth of Health Care Spending," January 2008.

25. Centers for Medicare and Medicaid Services, "National Health Expenditure Data for 1960–2013," Table 1.

26. Ibid.; Richard Kronick and Rosa Po,"Growth in Medicare Spending per Beneficiary Continues to Hit Historic Lows," ASPE Issue Brief, Office of the Assistant Secretary for Planning and Evaluation, Department of Health and Human Services, January 7, 2013.

27. Kronick and Po, "Growth in Medicare Spending."

28. *2014 Annual Report*, Table V.B.6.

29. Kaiser Family Foundation, "Key Issues in Understanding the Economic and Health Security of Current and Future Generations of Seniors," March 3, 2012.

30. Congressional Budget Office, "Reducing the Deficit: Spending and Revenue Options," Publication no. 4212, March 20, 2011.

31. *2014 Annual Report*, Table III.B.

32. C. Eugene Steurle and Caleb Quakenbush, "Social Security and Medicare Taxes and Benefits over a Lifetime: 2013 Update," Urban Institute, November 2013, http://www.urban.org/UploadedPDF/412945-Social-Security-and-Medicare-Taxes-and-Benefits-over-a-Lifetime.pdf.

33. *2014 Annual Report*," Figure II.E1.

34. Ibid.

35. That is the difference between Hospital Insurance payroll tax revenue and expenditures. *2014 Annual Report*, Table II.E1.

36. Social Security Administration, "Annual Statistical Supplement to the Social Security Bulletin, 2011," SSA Publication no. 13-11700, February 2012, Table 2.C1, http://www.ssa.gov/policy/docs/statcomps/supplement/2011/supplement11.pdf.

37. *2012 Annual Report of the Boards of Trustees of the Federal Hospital Insurance and Federal Supplementary Medical Insurance Trust Funds* (Baltimore: Centers for Medicare and Medicaid Services, April 23, 2012), Table II.F2, http://www.treasury.gov/resource-center/economic-policy/ss-medicare/Documents/TR_2012_Medicare.pdf.

38. *2014 Annual Report*, Table V.H6; Centers for Medicare and Medicaid Services, "National Health Expenditures; Aggregate and Per Capita Amounts, Annual Percent Change and Percent Distribution: Selected Calendar Years 1960–2013."

39. *2014 Annual Report*, Table IV.C2.

40. Ibid.

41. See Peter R. Orszag and Ezekiel J. Emanuel, "Health Care Reform and Cost Control," *New England Journal of Medicine* 363, no. 7 (August 2010): 601–3, http://www.nejm.org/doi/full/10.1056/NEJMp1006571.

42. Elmendorf , letter to the Honorable Nancy Pelosi on H.R. 4872.

43. Health Care and Education Affordability Reconciliation Act, Title I, Subtitle E, sec. 1411, and Subtitle A, sec. 9015.

44. Letter from Douglas Elmendorf, director, Congressional Budget Office, to the Honorable Harry Reid, December 19, 2009, http://www.cbo.gov/sites/default/files/cbofiles/ftpdocs/108xx/doc10868/12-19-reid_letter_managers_correction_noted.pdf.

45. Elmendorf, letter to the Honorable Nancy Pelosi on H.R. 4872.

46. "ACR Strongly Opposes Imaging Cuts in Health Care and Education Afford-ability Reconciliation Act," DOTmed, March 19, 2010, http://www.dotmed.com/news/story/12058/.

47. Elmendorf, letter to the Honorable Nancy Pelosi on H.R. 4872.

48. Patient Protection and Affordable Care Act, Title III, Subtitle B, Part III, sec. 3131.

49. Centers for Medicare and Medicaid Services, "Projected Medicare Expen-ditures under Illustrative Scenarios with Alternative Payment Updates to Medi-care Providers," May 18, 2012, http://www.cms.gov/Research-Statistics-Data-and-Systems/Statistics-Trends-and-Reports/ReportsTrustFunds/Downloads/2012TR AlternativeScenario.pdf.

50. Ibid.

51. Jonathan Skinner and Elliot S. Fisher, "Reflections on Geographic Variation in U.S. Health Care," Dartmouth Institute for Health Policy and Clinical Practice, March 31, 2010, http://www.dartmouthatlas.org/downloads/press/Skinner_Fisher_D A_05_10.pdf.

52. Ibid.

53. Out of 40 indicators studied. Steven M. Asch, Elizabeth M. Sloss, Christopher Hogan, Robert H. Brook, and Richard L. Kravitz, "Measuring Underuse of Necessary Care among Elderly Medicare Beneficiaries Using Inpatient and Outpatient Claims," *Journal of the American Medical Association* 284, no. 18 (November 8, 2000): 2325–33.

54. Daniel Polsky et al., "The Health Effects of Medicare for the Near-Elderly Uninsured," *Journal of Health Services Research* 44, no. 3 (June 2009):.

55. Amy Finkelstein and Robin McKnight, "What Did Medicare Do? The Initial Impact on Mortality and Out-of-Pocket Medical Spending," *Journal of Public Econom-ics* 92, no. 7 (July 2008).

56. Medicare Payment Advisory Commission, *Report to the Congress: Medicare Pay-ment Policy* (Washington: Government Printing Office, March 2014), p. 42, http://www.medpac.gov/documents/reports/mar14_entirereport.pdf?sfvrsn=0.

57. Barack Obama, State of the Union, Office of the Press Secretary, the White House, February 12, 2013, http://www.whitehouse.gov/the-press-office/2013/02/12/president-barack-obamas-state-union-address.

58. Author's calculations using figures from letter from Douglas W. Elmendorf, director, Congressional Budget Office, to the Honorable John Boehner on H.R. 6079, July 24, 2012, http://www.cbo.gov/sites/default/files/cbofiles/attachments/43471 -hr6079.pdf.

59. Office of Management and Budget, "The President's Budget for Fiscal Year 2015," Summary Tables: Table S-9, March 4, 2014, http://www.whitehouse.gov/sites/default/files/omb/budget/fy2015/assets/tables.pdf.

60. Centers for Medicare and Medicaid Services, "Projected Medicare Expendi-tures under Illustrative Scenarios."

61. Vivian Y. Wu, "Hospital Cost Shifting Revisited: New Evidence from the Bal-anced Budget Act of 1997," *International Journal of Health Care Finance and Economics* 10, no. 1 (2010): 61–83; Austin B. Frakt, "How Much Do Hospitals Cost Shift? A Review of the Evidence," *Milbank Quarterly* 89, no. 1 (March 2011): 90–130; Jack Zwanziger and Anil Bamezai, "Evidence of Cost Shifting in California Hospitals," *Health Affairs* 25, no. 1 (2006): 197–203, http://content.healthaffairs.org/content/25/1/197.full.

62. American Academy of Family Physicians, "Where Will Seniors Get Health Care?" news release, December 3, 2010, http://www.aafp.org/media-center/releases-statements/all/2010/medicare-cuts-2010.html.

63. American Medical Association, "Online Survey of Physicians: The Impact of Medicare Physician Payment on Seniors' Access to Care," May 2010, http://cathmed.org/assets/files/AMA,%20Participation%20in%20Medicare,%20May%20 2010.pdf.

64. Melinda Beck, "More Doctors Steer Clear of Medicare," *Wall Street Journal*, July 29, 2013, http://online.wsj.com/news/articles/SB1000142412788732397120457862615101724189.

65. Peter Whoriskey, Dan Keating, and Lena H. Sun, "Data Uncover Nation's Top Medicare Billers," *Washington Post*, April 9, 2014, http://www.washingtonpost.com/business/economy/data-uncover-nations-top-medicare-billers/2014/04/08/9101a77e-bf39-11e3-b574-f8748871856a_story.html; Centers for Medicare and Medicaid Services, "Medicare Provider Utilization and Payment Data: Physician and Other Supplier," 2014, http://www.cms.gov/Research-Statistics-Data-and-Systems/Statistics-Trends-and-Reports/Medicare-Provider-Charge-Data/Physician-and-Other-Supplier.html.

66. Patient Protection and Affordable Care Act, Title III, Subtitle C, sec. 3403.

67. To say that Congress has *never* cut Medicare spending is untrue. At least 11 times since 1980, Congress passed Medicare cuts that actually took place. Most were modest reductions in payments to certain types of providers, reductions in "disproportionate share" payments to hospitals or small increases in cost sharing by seniors or in Medicare premiums. At least in limited circumstances, Congress *has* been able to trim Medicare. However, major structural reforms have eluded Congress since the program's inception. See James Homey and Paul van de Water, "House-Passed and Senate Health Bills Reduce Deficit, Slow Health Costs, and Include Realistic Medicare Savings," Center on Budget and Policy Priorities, December 4, 2009.

68. Patient Protection and Affordable Care Act, Title III, Subtitle E, sec. 3403 (c)(2)(a)(ii).

69. Centers for Medicare and Medicaid Services, "Projected Medicare Expenditures under Illustrative Scenarios," Figure 2.

70. Richard S. Foster, chief actuary, Centers for Medicare and Medicaid Services, "The Estimated Effect of the Affordable Care Act on Medicare and Medicaid Outlays and Total National Health Care Expenditures," Testimony before the House Committee on the Budget, 112th Cong., 1st sess., January 26, 2011, http://budget.house.gov/uploadedfiles/fostertestimony1262011.pdf.

71. *2014 Annual Report*, Table V.D.I.

72. Ibid., Table V.G1.

73. Patient Protection and Affordable Care Act, Title X, Subtitle H, sec. 10906.

74. Aldona Robbins and Gary Robbins, "The Effect of the 1988 and 1990 Social Security Tax Increases," Institute for Research on the Economics of Taxation, 1991.

75. Congressional Budget Office, "Economic Effects of Policies Contributing to Fiscal Tightening in 2013," November 8, 2012, http://www.cbo.gov/sites/default/files/cbofiles/attachments/11-08-12-FiscalTightening.pdf.

76. J. P. Morgan, "The US Fiscal Cliff, an Update and a Downgrade," Economic Research Note, October 18, 2012, https://mm.jpmorgan.com/EmailPubServlet?h=c7s2j110&doc=GPS-965096-0.pdf. This effect is not confined to the United States. Researchers used a reform in Colombia that sharply increased payroll tax rates in

Colombia to examine the employment effects of payroll tax rates. They found that a 10 percent increase in payroll tax rates lowers employment by 4–5 percent. Adriana Kugler and Maurice Kugler, "Labor Market Effects of Payroll Taxes in Developing Countries: Evidence from Colombia," *Economic Development and Cultural Change* 57, no. 2 (2009): 335–58.

77. Bernhard Heitger, "The Impact of Taxation on Unemployment in OECD Countries," *Cato Journal* 22, no. 2 (Fall 2002): 333–54.

78. *The 2014 Annual Report of the Boards of Trustees of the Federal Hospital Insurance and Federal Supplementary Medical Insurance Trust Funds* (Baltimore: Centers for Medicare and Medicaid Services, July 28, 2014), Table V.E2, http://downloads.cms.gov /files/TR2014.pdf.

79. Centers for Medicare and Medicaid Services, "Medicare Statistical Supplement: 2012 Edition," Table 4.2, http://www.cms.gov/Research-Statistics-Data-and-Systems /Statistics-Trends-and-Reports/MedicareMedicaidStatSupp/Downloads/2012 _Section4.pdf#Table4.2.

80. Congressional Budget Office, "Options for Reducing the Deficit: 2014 to 2023," November 2013, http://www.cbo.gov/sites/default/files/cbofiles /attachments/44715-OptionsForReducingDeficit-3.

81. Karen Davis, Cathy Schoen, and Stuart Guterman, "Medicare Essential: An Option to Promote Better Care and Curb Spending Growth," *Health Affairs* 32, no. 5 (2013): 900–909, http://content.healthaffairs.Org/content/32/5/900.full.pdf+html; Robert A. Berenson and John Holahan, "Preserving Medicare: A Practical Approach to Controlling Spending," Urban Institute, September 2011. Note, these studies dealt with merging Parts A and B. They did not address the inclusion of Part D. However, the same logic would seem to apply.

82. Jackie Calmes and Robert Pear, "Talk of Medicare Changes Could Open Way to Budget Pact," *New York Times*, March 28, 2013, http://www.nytimes .com/2013/03/29/us/politics/common-ground-in-washington-for-medicare -changes.html?pagewanted=all.

83. National Commission on Fiscal Responsibility and Reform, "The Moment of Truth," December 1, 2010, http://www.fiscalcommission.gov/news/moment-truth -report-national-commission-fiscal-responsibility-and-reform.

84. Paul Ryan, "H.R. 6110: To Provide for the Reform of Health Care, the Social Security System, the Tax Code for Individuals and Business, and the Budget Process," 110th Cong., 2nd sess., May 21, 2008, http://www.gpo.gov/fdsys/pkg/BILLS-110hr6110ih /pdf/BILLS-110hr6110ih.pdf.

85. House Budget Committee, "The Path to Prosperity: Fiscal Year 2012 Budget Resolution," April 5, 2011, p. 46, http://budget.house.gov/uploadedfiles/pathtoprosperi tyfy2012.pdf.

86. House Budget Committee, "The Path to Prosperity: A Responsible, Balanced Budget, Fiscal Year 2014 Budget Resolution," March 2013, http://budget.house.gov /uploadedfiles/fy14budget.pdf.

87. Congressional Budget Office, "Options for Reducing the Deficit: 2014 to 2023."

88. Martin Feldstein, "Prefunding Medicare," *American Economic Review* 89, no. 2 (1999): 222–27.

89. Andrew J. Rettenmaier and Thomas R. Saving, "A Medicare Reform Proposal Everyone Can Love: Finding Common Ground among Medicare Reformers," NCPA Policy Report no. 306, National Center for Policy Analysis, December 2007.

90. Ibid.

91. Ibid.

Chapter 7

1. Congressional Budget Office, "Updated April Budget Projections—Medicaid Baseline Projections," April 14, 2014, http://www.cbo.gov/sites/default/files/cbofiles/attachments/44204-2014-04-Medicaid.pdf.

2. Department of Health and Human Services, "Federal Financial Participation in State Assistance Expenditures; Federal Matching Shares for Medicaid, the Children's Health Insurance Program, and Aid to Needy Aged, Blind, or Disabled Persons for October 1, 2012 through September 30, 2013," http://aspe.hhs.gov/health/reports/2013/FMAP2013/fmap2013.cfm.

3. Department of Health and Human Services, "2012 Actuarial Report on the Financial Outlook for Medicaid," http://www.medicaid.gov/Medicaid-CHIP-Program-Information/By-Topics/Financing-and-Reimbursement/Downloads/medicaid-actuarial-report-2012.pdf.

4. Ibid.

5. Kaiser Family Foundation, "Distribution of Medicaid Enrollees by Enrollment Group, FY2010," State Health Facts, http://kff.org/medicaid/state-indicator/distribution-by-enrollment-group/.

6. Department of Health and Human Services, "2012 Actuarial Report."

7. Ibid.

8. Congressional Budget Office, "Updated April Budget Projections—Medicaid."

9. Department of Health and Human Services, "2008 Actuarial Report on the Financial Outlook for Medicaid," https://www.cms.gov/Research-Statistics-Data-and-Systems/Research/ActuarialStudies/downloads/medicaidreport2008.pdf.

10. National Governors Association and National Association of State Budget Officers, "State Expenditure Report (Fiscal 2012-2014 Data)," http://www.nasbo.org/sites/default/files/State%20Expenditure%20Report%20%28Fiscal%202012-2014%29S.pdf.

11. *National Federation of Independent Business v. Sebelius*, 567 U.S. (2012).

12. Kaiser Family Foundation, "Current Status of State Medicaid Expansion Decisions," December 17, 2014.

13. Centers for Medicare and Medicaid Services, "Medicaid & CHIP: April 2014 Monthly Applications, Eligibility Determinations and Enrollment Report," Department of Health and Human Services, June 4, 2014. *Washington Post* fact checker Glenn Kessler gave this claim four Pinocchios for falsehood. Glenn Kessler, "Obama's Claim That 7 Million Got 'Access to Health Care for the First Time' Because of His Medicaid Expansion," *Washington Post*, February 24, 2014.

14. Congressional Budget Office, "Updated Estimates for the Insurance Coverage Provisions of the Affordable Care Act," March 13, 2012; Congressional Budget Office, "Effects on Health Insurance and the Federal Budget for the Insurance Coverage Provisions in the Affordable Care Act—April 2014 Baseline," April 14, 2014.

15. Ibid.

16. Sandra Decker, "In 2011 Nearly One-Third of Physicians Said They Would Not Accept New Medicaid Patients, but Rising Fees May Help," *Health Affairs* 31, no. 8 (2012): 1673–79.

17. Joanna Bisgaier and Karin V. Rhodes, "Auditing Access to Specialty Care for Children with Public Insurance," *New England Journal of Medicine* 364 (June 2011): 2324–33, http://www.nejm.org/doi/full/10.1056/NEJMsa1013285#t=articleTop.

18. Joanna Bisgaier, Diana B. Cutts, Burton L. Edelstein, and Karin V. Rhodes, "Disparities in Child Access to Emergency Care for Acute Oral Injury," *Pediatrics* 127, no. 6 (June 2011): 428–35.

19. Stephen Zuckerman, Laura Skopec, and Kristen McCormack, "Reversing the Medicaid Fee Bump: How Much Could Medicaid Physician Fees for Primary Care Fall in 2015," Urban Institute, Health Policy Center Brief, December 2014.

20. Damien J. LaPar et al., "Primary Payer Status Affects Mortality for Major Surgical Operations," *Annals of Surgery* 252, no. 3 (September 2010).

21. Jacques Hacquebord et al., "Medicaid Status Is Associated with Higher Complication Rates after Spine Surgery," *Spine* 38, no. 16 (July 2013): 1393–400; Seth A. Waits, Bradley N. Reames, Kyle H. Sheetz, Michael J. Englesbe, and Darrell A. Campbell, "Anticipating the Effects of Medicaid Expansion on Surgical Care," *JAMA Surgery* 149, no. 7 (2014): 745–47.

22. Katherine Baicker et al., "The Oregon Experiment—Medicaid's Effects on Clinical Outcomes," *New England Journal of Medicine* 368 (May 2013), http://www.nejm.org/doi/full/10.1056/NEJMsa1212321#t=article.

23. Centers for Medicare and Medicaid Services, "Medicaid & CHIP: April 2014 Monthly Applications, Eligibility Determinations and Enrollment Report."

24. Malcolm K. Sparrow, professor, John F. Kennedy School of Government, Harvard University, Testimony on "Criminal Prosecution as a Deterrent to Health Care Fraud" before the Subcommittee on Crime and Drugs of the Senate Committee on the Judiciary, 111th Cong., lst sess., "May 20, 2009, http://www.hks.harvard.edu/news-events/news/testimonies/sparrow-senate-testimony.

25. Daniel R. Levinson, inspector general, Department of Health and Human Services, Testimony on "Combating Fraud, Waste, and Abuse in Medicare and Medicaid," before the Senate Special Committee on Aging " 111th Cong., lst sess., May 6, 2009, http://www.hhs.gov/asl/testify/2009/05/t20090506d.html.

26. In particular, the Obama administration has advanced proposals to replace current federal matching rates, which vary depending on whether the recipient was eligible for Medicaid before the ACA expansion or as a result of that expansion, as well as for the Children's Health Insurance Program (CHIP), with a single "blended rate," which would effectively reduce the federal share of Medicaid funding, shifting more costs to the states. The administration initially anticipated approximately $100 billion in savings from that measure; in response to a lack of support, it subsequently attenuated the proposal in a subsequent budget, projecting only $18 billion in savings, and then dropped the blended rate altogether. Although it has been dropped from the president's annual budget, it remains one of the few significant cost-saving proposals that would keep Medicaid's current structure intact. The blended rate would leave the program essentially unchanged; its only effect would be to synthesize the different federal matching rates for the range of federal-state health programs (Medicaid, CHIP, the new Medicaid expansion population) into one "blended rate." Because this proposal does not change the program's structure, it does nothing to address its underlying problems and would achieve savings by merely shifting costs to the states. It has generated little support from either party, with Sen. Jay Rockefeller dismissing it as "not a viable option," and others pointing to the proposal as a reason to be wary of future federal cuts after states have committed to expanding their Medicaid programs.

27. This arrangement does not, of course, address the issue of preexisting conditions, since few insurers would be likely to accept Medicaid patients with such illnesses. However, most market-based reform proposals would address that issue separately, possibly through expanded use of subsidized "high-risk" pools.

28. The study did find some effect on mental health outcomes, as the researchers found that having Medicaid reduced the observed rates of depression by 30 percent. Medicaid did increase the probability of being diagnosed with depression, but it did not significantly increase the use of medication for depression. Baicker et al., "The Oregon Experiment."

29. Congressional Budget Office, "Updated April Budget Projections—Medicaid."

30. Congressional Budget Office, "Options for Reducing the Deficit: 2014 to 2023," Health Option 1, Function 550, November 13, 2013, http://www.cbo.gov/sites /default/files/cbofiles/attachments/44715-OptionsForReducingDeficit-3.pdf.

31. Congressional Budget Office, "Updated April Budget Projections—Medicaid."

32. House Budget Committee, "The Path to Prosperity: A Responsible, Balanced Budget, Fiscal Year 2014 Budget Resolution," March 2013, http://budget.house.gov /uploadedfiles/fy14budget.pdf.

Chapter 8

1. Charles Blahous, "The Unfolding Fiscal Disaster behind ACA Enrollment Figures," Mercatus Center, George Mason University, April 17, 2014, http://mercatus .org/expert_commentary/unfolding-fiscal-disaster-behind-aca-enrollment-Figures; Office of Management and Budget, "Historical Tables," April 24, 2014, Table 1.2, http://www.whitehouse.gov/omb/budget/historicals; Congressional Budget Office, "Updated Budget Projections: 2014 to 2024," April 14, 2014, http://www.cbo.gov /sites/default/files/cbofiles/attachments/45229-UpdatedBudgetProjections_2.pdf.

2. Blahous, "The Unfolding Fiscal Disaster."

3. The Patient Protection and Affordable Care Act and the Health Care and Education Affordability Reconciliation Act (HCEARA) combined have 2,562 pages and 511,520 words.

4. David Wessel, "Four Key Questions for Health-Care Law," *Wall Street Journal*, February 14, 2013, http://online.wsj.com/news/articles/SB1000142412788732443200 4578301854019979968.

5. Curtis W. Copeland, "New Entities Created Pursuant to the Patient Protection and Affordable Care Act," Congressional Research Service, July 8, 2010, https:// www.aamc.org/download/133856/data/crsentities.pdf.pdf.

6. Among provisions that have been postponed are (a) the employer mandate, (b) reporting requirements related to the employer mandate and subsidy determinations, (c) small business exchange (Small Business Health Options Program) enrollment, (d) out-of-pocket caps, (e) cuts to disproportionate share hospitals, and (f) the Basic Health Plan option. The administration has also extended the deadline for the closure of state high-risk pools and the deadline for health plans to comply with the essential health benefits in the law. Most recently, the administration exempted individuals whose policies have been canceled from the individual mandate.

7. Although most of the changes to the law have been enacted by the administration, some were passed by Congress. Most recently, the American Taxpayer Relief Act of 2012 officially repealed the Community Living Assistance Services and Supports

Act. The Middle Class Tax Relief and Job Creation Act of 2012 postponed cuts to hospitals that serve a disproportionate number of uninsured or underinsured patients. The Comprehensive 1099 Taxpayer Protection and Repayment of Exchange Subsidy Overpayments Act of 2011 repealed the requirement for businesses to file a Form 1099 whenever they pay a vendor more than $600 in a single year. C. Stephen Redhead and Janet Kinzer, "Legislative Actions to Repeal, Defund, or Delay the Affordable Care Act," Congressional Research Service, April 7, 2014, http://hr.cch.com/hld /CRSReportActionstoRepealACA.pdf.

8. Patient Protection and Affordable Care Act (Public Law 111-148), Title I, Subtitle F, Part I, sec. 1501, as amended by the Health Care and Education Affordability Reconciliation Act, sec. 1002. Note that this section amends Subtitle D of Chapter 48 of the Internal Revenue Code of 1986.

9. Ibid.

10. Patient Protection and Affordable Care Act, Title I, Subtitle D, sec. 1302(b)(l).

11. *National Federation of Independent Business v. Sebelius*, 567 U.S. (2012).

12. Roberts's ruling could also make it difficult to fix the adverse-selection problem should it develop. If the penalty for noncompliance was raised to a sufficiently coercive level that would make people buy insurance, by Roberts's logic, it would no longer be a tax but a mandate, something that he has said would be unconstitutional. In effect, Roberts has said that the ACA's individual mandate is constitutional precisely because it won't work.

13. Mark J. Mazur, "Continuing to Implement the ACA in a Careful, Thoughtful Manner," U.S. Treasury Department, July 2, 2013, http://www.treasury.gov/connect /blog/pages/continuing-to-implement-the-aca-in-a-careful-thoughtful-manner-.aspx.

14. U.S. Treasury Department, "Final Regulations Implementing Employer Shared Responsibility under the Affordable Care Act (ACA) for 2015," February 10, 2014.

15. Kaiser Family Foundation, "2013 Employer Health Benefits Survey," August 20, 2013, http://kff.org/private-insurance/report/2013-employer-health-benefits/.

16. Patient Protection and Affordable Care Act, Title I, Subtitle A, Part A, Subpart II, sec. 2714.

17. Ibid., Title 1, Subtitle A, Part A, Subpart II, sec. 2711. Before the passage of the Affordable Care Act, roughly 40 percent of insured Americans already had policies with no lifetime caps. For those policies that had a cap on lifetime benefits, that cap was usually somewhere between $2.5 million and $5 million, with many running as high as $8 million, amounts that very few people ever reached. Still, some individuals with chronic or catastrophic conditions will undoubtedly benefit from this provision, although there are no solid estimates on how many.

18. Public Health Service Act, Title XXVII, Part A, sec. 2712, as amended by the Patient Protection and Affordable Care Act, Title I, Subtitle A, sec. 1001.

19. Patient Protection and Affordable Care Act, Title IX, Subtitle A, sec. 9016(a).

20. Centers for Medicare and Medicaid Services, "80/20 Rule Delivers More Value to Consumers in 2012," http://www.cms.gov/CCIIO/Resources/Forms-Reports-and -Other-Resources/Downloads/2012-medical-loss-ratio-report.pdf.

21. Public Health Service Act, Title XXVII, Part A, sec. 2705(a)(l–9), as amended by the Patient Protection and Affordable Care Act, Title I, Subtitle C, sec. 1201.

22. Public Health Service Act, Title XXVII, Part A, sec. 2702(a), as amended by the Patient Protection and Affordable Care Act, Title I, Subtitle C, sec. 1201. The ban on medical underwriting may not be as effective as proponents hope in making insurance

available to those with preexisting conditions. Insurance companies have a variety of mechanisms for evading such restrictions. A simple example is for insurers to focus their advertising on young healthy people, or they can locate their offices on the top floor of a building with no elevator or provide free health club memberships while failing to include any oncologists in their network.

23. Public Health Service Act, Title XXVII, Part A, sec. 2701, as amended by the Patient Protection and Affordable Care Act, Title I, Subtitle C, sec. 1201.

24. Ibid., Title XXVII, Part A, sec. 2701(a)(l)(A)(iii), as amended.

25. Ibid., Title XXVII, Part A, sec. 2701(a)(l)(A)(iv), as amended.

26. Ibid., Title XXVII, Part A, sec. 2701(a)(l)(B), as amended.

27. Patient Protection and Affordable Care Act, Subtitle D, Part II, sec. 1311.

28. Kaiser Family Foundation, "State Health Insurance Marketplace Types, 2015," http://kff.org/health-reform/state-indicator/state-health-insurance-marketplace -types.

29. Amy Goldstein, "Obama Administration Prepares to Take Over Oregon's Broken Health Insurance Exchange," *Washington Post*, April 24, 2014, http:// www.washingtonpost.com/national/health-science/obama-administration -prepares-to-take-over-oregons-broken-health-insurance-exchange/2014/04/24 /ff9aa220-cbc4-11e3-95f7-7ecdde72d2ea_story.html.

30. Kaiser Family Foundation, "The Uninsured: A Primer—Key Facts about Health Insurance on the Eve of Coverage Expansions," October 23, 2013, http://kff.org /uninsured/report/the-uninsured-a-primer-key-facts-about-health-insurance-on -the-eve-of-coverage-expansions/.

31. Patient Protection and Affordable Care Act, Title II, Subtitle A, sec. 2002.

32. Ibid., Title II, Subtitle A, sec. 2001. The federal match rate is 100 percent through 2016, 95 percent for calendar quarters in 2017, 94 percent for calendar quarters in 2018, 93 percent for calendar quarters in 2019, and 90 percent thereafter.

33. Kaiser Family Foundation, "Current Status of State Medicaid Expansion Decisions," December 17, 2014.

34. Department of Health and Human Services, "Health Insurance Marketplace: Summary Enrollment Report for the Initial Annual Open Enrollment Period, For the Period: October 1, 2013–March 31, 2014 (Including Additional Special Enrollment Period Activity Reported through 4-19-14)," May 1, 2014, http://aspe.hhs.gov/health /reports/2014/MarketPlaceEnrollment/Apr2014/ib_2014apr_enrollment.pdf.

35. Office of the Assistant Secretary for Planning and Evaluation, "Health Insurance Marketplace 2015 Open Enrollment Period: December Enrollment Report," December 30, 2014.

36. Department of Health and Human Services, "Premium Affordability, Competi- tion, and Choice in the Health Insurance Marketplace, 2014," ASPE Research Brief, Department of Health and Human Services, June 18, 2014.

37. Congressional Budget Office, "Options for Reducing the Deficit: 2014 to 2023, Eliminate Exchange Subsidies for People with Income over 300 Percent of the Federal Poverty Guidelines," November 13, 2013.

38. Jonathan Adler and Michael Cannon, "The Halbig Cases: Desperately Seeking Ambiguity in Clear Statutory Text," *Journal of Health Politics* 40, no. 3 (November 25, 2014).

39. Michael Cannon, "The Flip-Flopping Architect of the ACA," *Politico Magazine*, July 28, 2014.

40. Congressional Budget Office, "Updated Estimates of the Effects of the Insurance Coverage Provisions of the Affordable Care Act, April 2014," April 14, 2014, http://www.cbo.gov/sites/default/files/cbofiles/attachments/45231-ACA_Estimates.pdf.

41. Letter from Douglas W. Elmendorf, director, Congressional Budget Office, to the Honorable Nancy Pelosi on H.R. 4872, the Reconciliation Act of 2010, March 20, 2010, https://www.cbo.gov/sites/default/files/cbofiles/ftpdocs/113xx/doc11379/amendreconprop.pdf.

42. Congressional Budget Office, "Updated Estimates, April 2014."

43. Congressional Budget Office, "Updated Budget Projections: 2014 to 2024"; Office of Management and Budget, "Historical Tables," April 24, 2014, Table 13.1, http://www.whitehouse.gov/omb/budget/historicals.

44. Letter from Douglas W. Elmendorf, director, Congressional Budget Office, to the Honorable John Boehner, February 18, 2011, http://www.cbo.gov/sites/default/files/cbofiles/ftpdocs/120xx/doc12069/hr2.pdf. It should be pointed out, however, that most of those authorizations—about $85 billion—were for activities that were already being carried out under prior law or that were previously authorized and that the ACA authorized for future years. Therefore, the repeal of those ACA authorizations would not necessarily result in discretionary savings of $100 billion for the 2012–2021 period.

45. Sam Baker, "Setup Costs Mount for ObamaCare Exchanges," *The Hill*, April 10, 2013, http://thehill.com/policy/healthcare/293071-costs-mount-for-health-laws-exchanges.

46. There is reason for skepticism about whether those savings will ever materialize. For example, the CBO has warned that many of the law's cost-saving provisions "might be difficult to sustain." Congressional Budget Office, "2013 Long-Term Budget Outlook," September 17, 2013. And Medicare's chief actuary also warned that projected savings "may be unrealistic." Richard S. Foster, *Estimated Financial Effects of the "Patient Protection and Affordable Care Act"* (Darby, PA: Diane Publishing, 2010), p. 8. However, for the sake of this analysis, we assume the savings will materialize.

47. *The 2010 Annual Report of the Board of Trustees of the Federal Old-Age and Survivors Insurance and Federal Disability Insurance Trust Fund* (Baltimore: Centers for Medicare and Medicaid Services, August 5, 2010), Table III.C15, http://www.socialsecurity.gov/OACT/TR/2010/tr10.pdf.

48. Perhaps the clearest explanation appeared in the Clinton administration's fiscal year 2000 budget, in reference to the Social Security Trust Fund: "These Trust Fund balances are available to finance future benefit payments … but only in a bookkeeping sense. … They do not consist of real economic assets that can be drawn down in the future to fund benefits. Instead, they are claims on the Treasury that, when redeemed, will have to be financed by raising taxes, borrowing from the public, or reducing benefits or other expenditures. The existence of Trust Fund balances, therefore, does not by itself have any impact on the government's ability to pay benefits." Executive Office of the President of the United States, *Analytic Perspectives: Budget of the United States Government, Fiscal Year 2000* (Washington: Government Printing Office, 1999), p. 337, http://www.gpo.gov/fdsys/pkg/BUDGET-2000-PER/pdf/BUDGET-2000-PER.pdf.

49. Foster, *Estimated Financial Effects of the Affordable Care Act*.

50. Author's calculations using Congressional Budget Office, "Updated Estimates, April 2014; letter from Douglas W. Elmendorf, director, Congressional Budget Office, to the Honorable John Boehner on H.R. 6079, July 24, 2012, http://www.cbo.gov/sites/default/files/cbofiles/attachments/43471-hr6079.pdf.

51. Ibid.

52. Patient Protection and Affordable Care Act, Title IX, Subtitle A, sec. 9001, as amended by the HCEARA, sec. 1401.

53. Foster, *Estimated Financial Effects of the Affordable Care Act*.

54. Towers Watson, "Cadillac Health Plan Tax to Penalize Majority of Employers by 2018," news release, May 19, 2010, http://www.towerswatson.com/en-US /Press/2010/05/Cadillac-Health-Plan-Tax-to-Penalize-Majority-of-Employers-by-2018.

55. Patient Protection and Affordable Care Act, Title IX, Subtitle A, sec. 9015.

56. Health Care and Education Affordability Reconciliation Act, Title I, Subtitle E, sec. 1411.

57. Patient Protection and Affordable Care Act, Title IX, Subtitle A, sec. 9013.

58. Ibid., Title IX, Subtitle A, sec. 9013(b).

59. Ibid., Title IX, Subtitle A, sec. 9008, as amended by the HCEARA, sec. 1404.

60. Ibid., Title IX, Subtitle A, sec. 9009, as amended by the HCEARA, sec. 1405.

61. Ibid., Title IX, Subtitle A, sec. 9009, as amended by the HCEARA, sec. 1405(b) (2)(E).

62. Foster, *Estimated Financial Effects of the Affordable Care Act*, p. 16.

63. "New Tax Could Boost Small Business Premiums by $1,000 per Year," Joint Economic Committee, Republican staff, April 22, 2010, http://heartland.org/sites /all/modules/custom/heartland_migration/files/pdfs/27697.pdf.

64. Patient Protection and Affordable Care Act, Subtitle A, sec. 9010, as amended by the HCEARA, sec. 1406(a)(4).

65. Ibid., Title IX, Subtitle A, sec. 9010, as amended by the HCEARA, sec. 1406.

66. Ibid., Title IX, Subtitle A, sec. 9010(b)(l)(A).

67. Ibid., Title IX Subtitle A, sec. 9010(c)(2)(C), as amended by Title X, Subtitle H, sec. 10905(c), and Subtitle A, sec. 9010(c)(2)(E), as amended by Title X, Subtitle H, sec. 10905(c).

68. Ibid., Title IX, Subtitle A, sec. 9010(c)(2)(C), as amended by Title X, Subtitle H, sec.10905(d). AARP insurance plans are also exempt from several other provisions of the law, including the prohibition on excluding preexisting conditions (sec. 1201[2][A]), medical loss ratio requirements (sec. 1103), and limits on compensation for insurance executives (sec. 9014).

69. Patrick Fleenor and Gerald Prante, "Health Care Reform: How Much Does It Redistribute Income?" Fiscal Fact no. 22, Tax Foundation, April 15, 2010, http://taxfoundation.org/article/health-care-reform-how-much-does-it -redistribute-income. That amount is on top of what was already expected to accrue to families in the top 1 percent of incomes.

70. Ibid. Those with incomes of less than $18,000 per year gain relatively little because they already receive government assistance under Medicaid and other programs.

71. Elmendorf, letter to the Honorable John Boehner, July 24, 2012.

72. Nila Ceci-Renaud and Paul-Antoine Chevalier, "L'impact des seuils de 10, 20 et 50 salariés sur la taille des entreprises françaises," *Économie et Statistique*, no. 437 (March 2011): 29–45, http://www.insee.fr/fr/ffc/docs_ffc/es437b.pdf.

73. Dennis Jacobe, "Half of U.S. Small Businesses Think Health Law Bad for Them," Gallup, May 10, 2013, http://www.gallup.com/poll/162386/half-small -businesses-think-health-law-bad.aspx.

74. Bill McInturff and Micah Roberts, "Presentation of Findings from National Research Conducted among Business Decision-Makers: September–October 2013," U.S. Chamber

of Commerce and International Franchise Association, October 2013, p. 4, https://www
.uschamber.com/sites/default/files/legacy/reports/IFAChamberFinal.pdf.

75. Jacobe, "Half of U.S. Small Businesses Think Health Law Bad for Them."

76. Ben Casselman, "Yes, Some Companies Are Cutting Hours in Response
to 'Obamacare,'" *FiveThirtyEight*, January 13, 2015, http://fivethirtyeight.com
/features/yes-some-companies-are-cutting-hours-in-response-to-obamacare.

77. Ibid.

78. Kaiser Family Foundation, "2013 Employer Health Benefits Survey, Percentage
of Firms Offering Health Benefits, by Firm Size, 1999–2013," August 20, 2013.

79. Diana Furchtgott-Roth and Harold Furchtgott-Roth, "Employment Effects
of the New Excise Tax on the Medical Device Industry," September 2011, http://
www.chi.org/uploadedFiles/Industry_at_a_glance/090711EmploymentEffectofT
axonMedicalDeviceIndustryFINAL.pdf.

80. Michael J. Chow, "Effects of the ACA Health Insurance Premium Tax on Small
Businesses and Their Employees: An Update," National Federation of Independent
Business, March 19, 2013.

81. Andrew Lundeen, "Obamacare Tax Increases Will Impact Us All," Tax Foundation, March 5, 2013, http://taxfoundation.org/blog/obamacare-tax-increases
-will-impact-us-all.

82. Staff at the Ways and Means, Education and the Workforce, and Energy and
Commerce Committees, "Obamacare Burden Tracker," February 2013, http://
waysandmeans.house.gov/uploadedfiles/aca_burden_tracker_.pdf.

83. Chris Conover, "Congress Should Account for the Excess Burden of Taxation," Cato Institute Policy Analysis no. 669, October 13, 2010, http://www.cato
.org/sites/cato.org/files/pubs/pdf/PA669.pdf; Chris Conover, "Healthcare Law
Will Cost 1 Million or More Jobs," *Forbes*, July 31, 2012, http://www.forbes.com
/sites/chrisconover/2012/07/31/healthcare-law-will-cost-1-million-or-more-jobs.

84. Congressional Budget Office, "Labor Market Effects of the Affordable Care
Act: Updated Estimates," April 14, 2014, http://www.cbo.gov/sites/default
/files/cbofiles/attachments/45010-breakout-AppendixC.pdf.

85. Congressional Budget Office, "The Budget and Economic Outlook: 2014
to 2024," February 2014, http://www.cbo.gov/sites/default/files/cbofiles
/attachments/45010-Outlook2014_Feb.pdf.

86. Avik Roy, "49-State Analysis: Obamacare to Increase Individual-Market
Premiums by Average of 41%," *Forbes*, November 4, 2013, http://www.forbes
.com/sites/theapothecary/2013/11/04/49-state-analysis-obamacare-to-increase
-individual-market-premiums-by-avg-of-41-subsidies-flow-to-elderly/.

87. Office of the Assistant Secretary for Planning and Evaluation, "Health Insurance Marketplace Premiums for 2014," ASPE Issue Brief, Department of Health and
Human Services, September 25, 2013, http://aspe.hhs.gov/health/reports/2013
/marketplacepremiums/ib_marketplace_premiums.cfm.

88. Ibid.

89. Centers for Medicare and Medicaid Services, "Where Federal Health Exchange
Rates Will Rise," *New York Times*, November 14, 2014, http://www.nytimes.com
/interactive/2014/11/14/us/Where-Federal-Health-Exchange-Rates-Will-Rise.html.

90. Kaiser Family Foundation, "Analysis of 2015 Premium Changes in the Affordable Care Act's Health Insurance Marketplaces," January 6, 2015.

91. Express Scripts, "First Look: Health Exchange Medication Utilization," April 9, 2014, http://lab.express-scripts.com/insights/government-programs/first-look-health-exchange-medication-utilization.

92. Gallup, "Newly Insured in 2014 Represent about 4% of U.S. Adults," April 16, 2014, http://www.gallup.com/poll/168548/newly-insured-2014-represent-adults.aspx.

93. Office of the Assistant Secretary for Planning and Evaluation, "Health Insurance Marketplace: Summary Enrollment Report"; Katherine Restrepo and Chris Conover, "Obamacare's Longshot: Assessing the Exchange Enrollment Derby," *Forbes*, May 5, 2014, http://www.forbes.com/sites/theapothecary/2014/05/05/obamacares-longshot/.

94. Restrepo and Conover, "Obamacare's Longshot."

95. Office of the Assistant Secretary for Planning and Evaluation, "Health Insurance Marketplace 2015 Open Enrollment Period: December Enrollment Report," December 30, 2014.

96. Brett O'Hara and Kyle Caswell, "Health Status, Health Insurance, and Medical Services Utilization: 2010," U.S. Census Bureau, July 2013, http://www.census.gov/prod/2012pubs/p70-133.pdf.

97. Ibid.

98. Department of Health and Human Services, "Patient Protection and Affordable Care Act: HHS Notice of Benefit and Payment Parameters for 2015," final rule, *Federal Register*, March 11, 2014, https://www.federalregister.gov/articles/2014/03/11/2014-05052/patient-protection-and-affordable-care-act-hhs-notice-of-benefit-and-payment-parameters-for-2015. Congress included an amendment in the 2015 omnibus budget appropriations bill that tried to ensure that only fees could be used to pay insurers and prevented CMS from using other funds. This, to some extent, ensures taxpayers will not have to bail out insurers if the user fees do not prove sufficient. Section 227 provides that CMS may not transfer other funds from other accounts to pay for the risk corridor program. The CMS program appropriation section, however, does appropriate user fees, which can therefore be used to fund the risk corridor program. Expenditures on the program, however, cannot exceed the funds collected. Timothy Jost, "Implementing Health Reform: Open Enrollment Progress for 2015," *Health Affairs* (blog), December 31, 2014, http://healthaffairs.org/blog/2014/12 /12/implementing-health-reform-beneath-the-hood-of-the-cromnibus.

99. That is not to say that the government's stated goal of providing something approximating universal coverage is an unalloyed good. There are many concerns as to whether that is a proper responsibility of government. Even if one thinks government has some responsibility to subsidize medical care for those who cannot afford it, it is unclear that mandating health care insurance is the best method to do so, as opposed to tax credits or direct cash payment, for example. However, given that the ACA is current law and will intervene in the market in myriad ways, it can still be hoped that it would be relatively effective or efficient in pursuing that goal. As it stands, that amount of distortion and disruption is an incredibly high price to pay for the law's relatively small (compared with stated goals) increase in insurance coverage. In other words, there is little "bang for the buck."

100. Elmendorf, letter to the Honorable Nancy Pelosi, March 20, 2010.

101. Congressional Budget Office, "Updated Estimates, April 2014." Note the totals do not add up completely because of some shifting and churn.

102. Ibid.

103. Office of the Assistant Secretary for Planning and Evaluation, "How Many Individuals Might Have Marketplace Coverage After the 2015 Open Enrollment Period," Department of Heath and Human Services, November 10, 2014.

104. Sara R. Collins, Petra W. Rasmussen, and Michelle Doty, "Gaining Ground: Americans' Health Insurance Coverage and Access to Care After the Affordable Care Act's First Open Enrollment Period," The Commonwealth Fund, July 10, 2014.

105. There is not a reliable estimate for the previously uninsured rate of new Medicaid enrollees in the second round of open enrollment. This calculation uses the rate the Commonwealth Fund found from the first year of open enrollment and the most recent Medicaid enrollment data available. Author's calculations using Sara R. Collins, Petra W. Rasmussen, and Michelle Doty, "Gaining Ground"; Centers for Medicare and Medicaid Services, "Medicaid & CHIP: March 2014 Monthly Applications, Eligibility Determinations, and Enrollment Report," Department of Health and Human Services, May 1, 2014, http://www.medicaid.gov/AffordableCareAct/Medicaid-Moving-Forward-2014/Downloads/March-2014-Enrollment-Report.pdf.

106. Ibid.

107. Congressional Budget Office, "Updated Estimates, April 2014."

108. Barack Obama, "Remarks by the President at the Annual Conference of the American Medical Association," Office of the Press Secretary, the White House, June 15, 2009, http://www.whitehouse.gov/the-press-office/remarks-president-annual-conference-american-medical-association.

109. Barack Obama, interview by Chuck Todd, NBC News, November 7, 2013, http://www.nbcnews.com/video/nbc-news/53492840#53492840.

110. Lisa Myers, "Insurers, State Officials Say Cancellation of Health Care Policies Just as They Predicted," NBC News, November 15, 2013, http://www.nbcnews.com/news/other/insurers-state-officials-say-cancellation-health-care-policies-just-they-f2D 11603425.

111. Ibid.

112. Obama, interview.

113. Patient Protection and Affordable Care Act, Title I, Subtitle F, Part I, sec. 1501.

114. Ibid., Title I, Subtitle C, Part D, sec. 1251.

115. Department of Health and Human Services, "Group Health Plans and Health Insurance Coverage Relating to Status as a Grandfathered Health Plan under the Patient Protection and Affordable Care Act," interim final rule and proposed rule, *Federal Register*, June 17, 2010.

116. Center for Consumer Information and Insurance Oversight, "Letter to Insurance Commissioners," Centers for Medicare and Medicaid Services, November 14, 2013, http://www.cms.gov/CCIIO/Resources/Letters/Downloads/commissioner-letter-11-14-2013.PDF.

117. California only allows extensions in the small group market. Oregon decided to allow renewals last year but has not decided whether to allow them to continue beyond 2015. Kevin Lucia, Katie Keith, and Sabrina Corlette, "Update: State Decisions on the Health Insurance Policy Cancellations Fix," Commonwealth Fund, January 8, 2014, http://www.commonwealthfund.org/publications/blog/2013/nov/state-decisions-on-policy-cancellations-fix.

118. Centers for Medicare and Medicaid Services, "Insurance Standards Bulletin Series—Extension of Transitional Policy through October 1, 2016," March 5, 2014, http://www.cms.gov/CCIIO/Resources/Regulations-and-Guidance/Downloads /transition-to-compliant-policies-03-06-2015.pdf.

119. Obama, interview.

120. David Firestone, "The Uproar over Insurance 'Cancellation' Letters," *New York Times*, October 30, 2013, http://takingnote.blogs.nytimes.com/2013/10/30/the-uproar -over-insurance-cancellation-letters/. In reality, virtually all insurance plans cover hospitalization, although some might cap reimbursements.

121. HealthPocket Inc., "Almost No Existing Health Plans Meet New ACA Essential Health Benefit Standards," March 7, 2013, http://www.healthpocket.com/healthcare -research/infostat/few-existing-health-plans-meet-new-aca-essential-health-benefit -standards/#.U3UCsygk 1Y.

122. Ibid.

123. Ibid.

124. Patient Protection and Affordable Care Act, Title I, Subtitle C, Part II, sec. 1251; Bernadette Fernandez, "Grandfathered Health Plans under the Patient Protection and Affordable Care Act (ACA)," Congressional Research Service, April 27, 2010, http:// www.ncsl.org/documents/health/grandfathered.pdf.

125. Kaiser Family Foundation, "Employer Health Benefits: 2013 Annual Survey," Section 13–Grandfathered Plans, August 20, 2013, http://kaiserfamilyfoundation. files.wordpress.com/2013/08/8465-employer-health-benefits-20131.pdf.

126. Avik Roy, "Obama Officials in 2010: 93 Million Americans Will Be Unable to Keep Their Health Plans under Obamacare," *Forbes*, October 31, 2013, http://www .forbes.com/sites/theapothecary/2013/10/31/obama-officials-in-2010-93-million -americans-will-be-unable-to-keep-their-health-plans-under-obamacare/.

127. Fernandez, "Grandfathered Health Plans."

128. Ibid.

129. Department of Health and Human Services, "Group Health Plans and Health Insurance Coverage," Table 3.

130. Ibid.

131. Medical Group Management Association, "Legislative and Executive Advocacy Response Network ACA Insurance Exchange Implementation," September 2013.

132. Cited by Robert Pear, "Lower Health Insurance Premiums to Come at Cost of Fewer Choices," *New York Times*, September 22, 2013, http://www.nytimes .com/2013/09/23/health/lower-health-insurance-premiums-to-come-at-cost-of -fewer-choices.html?pagewanted=all.

133. Ricardo Alonso-Zaldivar, "New Health Plans Sold through Exchanges Not Accepted at Some Prestigious New York Hospitals," Associated Press, November 20, 2013.

134. Anna Wilde Mathews, "Many Health Insurers to Limit Choices of Doctors, Hospitals," *Wall Street Journal*, August 14, 2013, http://online.wsj.com/news/articles /SB10001424127887323446404579010800462478682.

135. Richard Cowart, "ACA Health Plan May Not Include Your Doctor," *Tennessean*, August 21, 2013, http://archive.tennessean.com/article/20130821 /BUSINESS/308210064/Richard-Cowart-ACA-health-plan-may-not-include-your -doctor.

136. Ben Leubsdorf, "Anthem Takes Heat from N.H. Senators over Limited Provider Network for Marketplace Plans," *Concord Monitor*, September 19, 2013, http://www.concordmonitor.com/news/work/business/8491779-95/anthem-takes-heat-from-nh-senators-over-limited-provider-network-for-marketplace-plans.

137. Sandhya Somashekhar and Ariana Eunjung Cha, "Insurers Restricting Choice of Doctors and Hospitals to Keep Costs Down," *Washington Post*, November 20, 2013, http://www.washingtonpost.com/national/health-science/insurers-restricting-choice-of-doctors-and-hospitals-to-keep-costs-down/2013/11/20/98c84e20-4bb4-11e3-ac54-aa84301ced81_story.html.

138. Ibid.

139. Christopher Weaver and Melinda Beck, "Insurers Cut Doctors Fees in New Plans," *Wall Street Journal*, November 15, 2013, http://online.wsj.com/news/articles/SB10001424052702304607104579212450545926912.

140. Unpublished McKinsey & Company study, cited by Mathews, "Many Health Insurers to Limit Choices."

141. Carl Campanile, "Out-of-Network Not an Option in Individual ObamaCare Plans," *New York Post*, October 23, 2012, http://nypost.com/2013/10/23/out-of-network-not-an-option-in-individual-obamacare-plans/.

142. "ObamaCare Architect: If You Like Your Doctor, You Can Pay More," *Fox News Sunday*, December 8, 2013, http://nation.foxnews.com/2013/12/08/obamacare-architect-if-you-your-doctor-you-can-pay-more.

143. Deloitte Center for Health Solutions, "Deloitte 2013 Survey of U.S. Physicians, Physician Perspectives About Health Care Reform and the Future of the Medical Profession," March 2014.

144. Physicians Foundation, "A Survey of America's Physicians: Practice Patterns and Perspectives," September 21, 2012, http://www.physiciansfoundation.org/healthcare-research/a-survey-of-americas-physicians-practice-patterns-and-perspectives/.

145. Richard Pollock, "Doctors Boycotting California's Obamacare Exchange," *Washington Examiner*, December 6, 2013, http://washingtonexaminer.com/doctors-boycotting-californias-obamacare-exchange/article/2540272.

146. Physicians Foundation, "Survey of America's Physicians."

147. Association of American Medical Colleges, "Physician Shortages to Worsen without Increases in Residency Training," September 30, 2010, https://www.aamc.org/download/150584/data/physician_shortages_factsheet.pdf.

148. World Bank, "Physicians (per 1,000 People)," Databank, http://data.worldbank.org/indicator/SH.MED.PHYS.ZS.

149. Clara Ritger, "Obama's Affordable Care Act Looking a Bit Unaffordable," *National Journal*, August 29, 2013, http://www.nationaljournal.com/domesticpolicy/obama-s-affordable-care-act-looking-a-bit-unaffordable-20130829.

150. Department of Labor, "FAQs about Affordable Care Act Implementation Part XII," February 2013, http://www.dol.gov/ebsa/faqs/faq-aca12.html.

151. Douglas W. Elmendorf, director, Congressional Budget Office, "CBO's Analysis of the Major Health Care Legislation Enacted in March 2010," Testimony before the Subcommittee on Health of the House Committee on Energy and Commerce, 112th Cong., 1st sess., March 30, 2011.

152. Center Forward, "Impact Analyses in Six States of the Patient Protection and Affordable Care Act (ACA)," May 2013, http://center-forward.org/wp-content/uploads/2013/05/ACA-Impact-Analysis-Executive-Summary.pdf.

153. House Committee on Energy and Commerce, "The Looming Premium Rate Shock," May 13, 2013, http://energycommerce.house.gov/sites/republicans .energycommerce.house.gov/files/analysis/insurancepremiums/FinalReport.pdf.

154. Among fully insured firms, so this excludes self-insured large firms. Kaiser Family Foundation and Health Research and Educational Trust, "Employer Health Benefits, 2014 Annual Survey," September 10, 2014.

155. Robert B. Helms, "Tax Policy and the History of the Health Insurance Industry," paper presented at "Taxes and Health Insurance: Analysis and Policy" Conference sponsored by the Tax Policy Center and the American Tax Policy Institute, Brookings Institution, Washington, DC, February 29, 2008, http://www .americantaxpolicyinstitute.org/pdf/health_conference/Helms.pdf.

156. Joseph P. Newhouse et al., "Some Interim Results from a Controlled Trial of Cost Sharing in Health Insurance," *New England Journal of Medicine* 305 (December 1981): 1501–7. See also Willard G. Manning et al., "Health Insurance and the Demand for Medical Care: Evidence from a Randomized Experiment," *American Economic Review* 77, no. 3 (1987): 251–73.

157. Liran Einave et al., "Selection on Moral Hazard in Health Insurance," *American Economic Review* 103, no. 1 (2013): 178–219, http://economics.mit.edu/files/7870.

158. *Burwell v. Hobby Lobby Stores, Inc.* 573 U.S. (2014).

159. Internal Revenue Service, "Health Savings Accounts and Other Tax Favored Health Plans," Publication 969.

160. Devon M. Harrick, "How to Create a Competitive Insurance Market," National Center for Policy Analysis, June 15, 2006, http://www.ncpa.org/pub/ba558.

161. Sue A. Blevins, "The Medical Monopoly: Protecting Consumers or Limiting Competition?" Cato Institute Policy Analysis no. 246, December 15, 1995.

162. Barack Obama, "Remarks by the President in Town Hall Meeting on Health Care," Office of the Press Secretary, the White House, June 11, 2009, http://www .whitehouse.gov/the_press_office/Remarks-by-the-President-in-Town-Hall-Meeting -on-Health-Care-in-Green-Bay-Wisconsin.

Chapter 9

1. Margaret Thatcher, interview by Llew Gardner, Thames TV *This Week*, February 5, 1976, http://www.margaretthatcher.org/speeches/displaydocument .asp?docid= 102953.

2. On average, a college student today will graduate with a debt of $29,400. Institute for College Access and Success, "The Project on Student Debt," 2013, http:// projectonstudentdebt.org/state_by_state-data.php.

3. Congressional Budget Office, "2013 Long-Term Budget Outlook," September 17, 2013, http://www.cbo.gov/sites/default/files/cbofiles/attachments/45308-2013-09 -LTBOSuppData.xlsx.

4. It's also worth pointing out that the top 1 percent earns 16 percent of all income in the United States but pays 36.7 percent of all federal income taxes. In fact, the 400 richest Americans together pay nearly as much in federal income taxes as do the 50 percent of taxpayers at the low end of the scale. The current tax code is already highly progressive. The wealthy pay a far higher effective tax rate. After all deductions and exemptions are included, the rich pay roughly 24 percent of their income in

taxes, compared with 11 percent on average for all taxpayers. The rich, it would seem, already pay more than their "fair share."

5. Office of Management and Budget, "The President's Budget for Fiscal Year 2015," Summary Tables: Table S-2, March 4, 2014, http://www.whitehouse.gov /sites/default/files/omb/budget/fy2015/assets/tables.pdf.

6. Office of Management and Budget, "Historical Tables," April 24, 2014, Table 3.2, http://www.whitehouse.gov/omb/budget/historicals.

7. Planned Parenthood, "Annual Report 2012–2013," p. 18, http://www.planned parenthood.org/files/7413/9620/1089/AR-FY13_111213_vF_rev3_ISSUU.pdf; Corporation for Public Broadcasting, "Fiscal Year 2014 Operating Budget," September 11, 2013, http://www.cpb.org/aboutcpb/financials/budget/FY2014-Operating-Budget.pdf.

8. Congressional Budget Office, "Updated Budget Projections: 2014 to 2024," April 2014, http://www.cbo.gov/sites/default/files/cbofiles/attachments/45229 -UpdatedBudgetProjections_2.pdf.

9. Jonathan Allen and Tony Capaccio, "Obama Said to Seek 7% Budget Boost, Setting Up Fight With Congress," Bloomberg Politics, January 15, 2015.

10. Congressional Budget Office, "An Update to the Budget and Economic Outlook: 2014 to 2024," August 27, 2014.

11. House Budget Committee, "The Path to Prosperity: Fiscal Year 2015 Budget Resolution," April 2014, http://budget.house.gov/uploadedfiles/fy15_blueprint .pdf. This budget is helped by $175 billion in "macroeconomic effects" that lower cumulative deficits by that amount over the period, because Ryan et al. assume lower spending, debt, and taxes will have positive macroeconomic effects. That assumption is not really that controversial, but most budgets use static scoring, and quantifying those effects can be tricky.

12. Allen and Capaccio, "Obama Said to Seek 7% Budget Boost."

13. Congressional Budget Office, "Updated Budget Projections: 2014 to 2024."

14. The 2014 Annual Report of the Board of Trustees of the Federal Old-Age and Survivors Insurance and Federal Disability Insurance Trust Fund (Washington: Government Printing Office, July 28, 2013), http://www.ssa.gov/oact/tr/2014/tr2014.pdf.

15. *The 2009 Annual Report of the Boards of Trustees of the Federal Hospital Insurance and Federal Supplementary Medical Insurance Trust Funds* (Baltimore: Centers for Medicare and Medicaid Services, May 12, 2009), https://www.cms.gov /Research-Statistics-Data-and-Systems/Statistics-Trends-and-Reports/Reports TrustFunds/downloads/tr2009.pdf.

16. *2014 Annual Report.*

17. Congressional Budget Office, "Updated Budget Projections: 2014 to 2024."

18. Ibid.

19. Congressional Budget Office, "The 2013 Long-Term Budget Outlook," September 17, 2013, http://www.cbo.gov/sites/default/files/cbofiles/attachments/44521 -LTBO2013_0.pdf.

20. Robert Frost, "The Road Not Taken," accessed via Poetry Foundation, http:// www.poetryfoundation.org/poem/173536.

Index

Page references followed by t or f indicate tables and figures, respectively.

About the Author

Michael Tanner is a senior fellow with the Cato Institute, where he heads research into a variety of domestic policies, with a particular emphasis on poverty, social welfare policy, health care reform, and Social Security. Under Tanner's direction, Cato launched the Project on Social Security Choice, which is widely considered the leading impetus for transforming the soon-to-be-bankrupt system into a private savings program. *Time* magazine calls Tanner "one of the architects of the private accounts movement," and *Congressional Quarterly* named him one of the nation's five most influential experts on Social Security.

He is also the author of numerous books on public policy, including *Leviathan on the Right: How Big-Government Conservatism Brought Down the Republican Revolution; Healthy Competition: What's Holding Back Health Care and How to Free It; The Poverty of Welfare: Helping Others in Civil Society;* and *A New Deal for Social Security.* Tanner's writings have appeared in nearly every major American newspaper, including the *New York Times,* the *Washington Post,* the *Los Angeles Times,* the *Wall Street Journal,* and *USA Today.* He writes a weekly column for *National Review Online,* and is a contributing columnist with the *New York Post.* A prolific writer and frequent guest lecturer, Tanner appears regularly on network and cable news programs. The *New York Times* refers to him as "a lucid writer and skilled polemicist."

Cato Institute

Founded in 1977, the Cato Institute is a public policy research foundation dedicated to broadening the parameters of policy debate to allow consideration of more options that are consistent with the principles of limited government, individual liberty, and peace. To that end, the Institute strives to achieve greater involvement of the intelligent, concerned lay public in questions of policy and the proper role of government.

The Institute is named for Cato's Letters, libertarian pamphlets that were widely read in the American Colonies in the early 18th century and played a major role in laying the philosophical foundation for the American Revolution.

Despite the achievement of the nation's Founders, today virtually no aspect of life is free from government encroachment. A pervasive intolerance for individual rights is shown by government's arbitrary intrusions into private economic transactions and its disregard for civil liberties. And while freedom around the globe has notably increased in the past several decades, many countries have moved in the opposite direction, and most governments still do not respect or safeguard the wide range of civil and economic liberties.

To address those issues, the Cato Institute undertakes an extensive publications program on the complete spectrum of policy issues. Books, monographs, and shorter studies are commissioned to examine the federal budget, Social Security, regulation, military spending, international trade, and myriad other issues. Major policy conferences are held throughout the year, from which papers are published thrice yearly in the Cato Journal. The Institute also publishes the quarterly magazine Regulation.

In order to maintain its independence, the Cato Institute accepts no government funding. Contributions are received from foundations, corporations, and individuals, and other revenue is generated from the sale of publications. The Institute is a nonprofit, tax-exempt, educational foundation under Section 501(c)3 of the Internal Revenue Code.

CATO INSTITUTE
1000 Massachusetts Ave., N.W.
Washington, D.C. 20001
www.cato.org